Managing Strokes and TIAs

in Practice

Ronald S MacWalter

Stroke Studies Centre, University Department
of Medicine, Ninewells Hospital and Medical
School, Dundee, UK

Colin P Shirley

Stroke Studies Centre, University Department
of Medicine, Ninewells Hospital and Medical
School, Dundee, UK

© 2003 Royal Society of Medicine Press Ltd
Published by the Royal Society of Medicine Press Ltd
1 Wimpole Street, London W1G 0AE, UK
Tel: +44 (0)20 7290 2921
Fax: +44 (0)20 7290 2929
Email: publishing@rsm.ac.uk
Website: www.rsmpress.co.uk

British library cataloguing in publication data
A catalogue record for this book is available from the British Library

ISBN 1-85315-517-9

ISSN 1473-6845

Distribution in Europe and Rest of World:
Marston Book Services Ltd
PO Box 269
Abingdon
Oxon OX14 4YN, UK
Tel: +44 (0)1235 465500
Fax: +44 (0)1235 465555

Distribution in the USA and Canada:
Jamco Distribution Inc
1401 Lakeway Drive
Lewisville, TX 75057, USA
Tel: +1 800 538 1287
Fax: +1 972 353 1303.
Email: jamco@majors.com

Distribution in Australia and New Zealand:
MacLennan + Petty Pty Ltd
Suite 405, 152 Bunnerong Road
Eastgardens NSW 2036
Australia
Tel: +61 2 9349 5811
Fax: +61 2 9349 5911

Phototypeset by Phoenix Photosetting, Chatham, Kent
Printed in Great Britain by Latimer Trend & Company Ltd, Plymouth

About the authors

Ronald S MacWalter BMSc (Hons) MD FRCP (Edin) FRCP (Glas)

Dr Ronald MacWalter is Consultant Physician in general medicine and acute stroke medicine at Ninewells Hospital and Medical School, Dundee and Honorary Senior Lecturer in medicine at the University of Dundee. He is also Honorary Associate Professor of medicine at the Kigezi International School of Medicine, Cambridge, England. He trained in Dundee and Oxford and developed a clinical and research interest in stroke and its management. He is a member of the British Association of Stroke Physicians, the British Hypertension Society and the British Geriatrics Society, and an executive committee member of the Scottish Heart & Arterial Risk Prevention group (SHARP). He has developed a number of guidelines for stroke patients and chaired the Scottish Intercollegiate Guidelines Network development group on hypertension in older people. His particular interests include acute treatment of stroke, rehabilitation and the prognosis of patients with stroke.

Colin P Shirley MB ChB (Hons) MRCP (UK)

Dr Colin Shirley is a Research Associate in stroke and is continuing to develop his career before taking up a consultant post. He has considerable expertise in the management and rehabilitation of acute stroke patients.

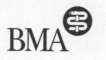

Preface

Stroke and transient ischaemic attack (TIA) are often neglected illnesses. They are a major cause of death and disability and must be treated as an emergency. We outline the various stages in the management of stroke and TIA in this book. The book aims to provide a practical guide for the busy clinician and is important in the treatment of patients and in the secondary prevention of stroke where there have been great developments over the past 10 years.

RS MacWalter
CP Shirley

Acknowledgements

We are grateful to our friend and colleague Dr Sarah Zahia for her valued comments and suggestions. We are grateful to Dr Sheila Nicoll and Dr Ann Shilton for their ongoing forbearance. We also thank Dr Andy Muir and all our other colleagues for their many valuable suggestions.

Contents

Introduction

Stroke is a syndrome characterized by 'rapidly developing clinical signs of focal (or global) disturbance lasting 24 hours or longer or leading to death with no apparent cause other than of vascular origin'. Stroke is a very important illness. When stroke and ischaemic heart disease are considered together, they constitute the leading cause of death in the world. When the burdens of disability and death are taken into account, stroke, which is already an important condition globally, will assume an even more important place in the future than it does at present. On its own, stroke is the third most common cause of death in the developed world after ischaemic heart disease and cancer.

> Stroke is the third most common cause of death in the developed world, but is the leading cause when considered along with ischaemic heart disease

Transient ischaemic attacks (TIAs) can be defined as episodes of focal loss of cerebral or monocular function due to embolic or thrombotic vascular disease lasting less than 24 hours.

The World Health Organization international classification of impairment, disabilities and handicaps provides the following framework for considering the impact of stroke on the individual:

- pathology (disease or diagnosis) – operating at the level of the organ or organ system
- impairment (symptoms and signs) – operating at the level of the whole body
- activity (disability) – observed behaviour or function
- participation (handicap) – social position and roles of the individual.

This framework can be affected by a number of contextual factors including personal experiences (eg previous illness), physical environment (house and local environment) and social environment (social network and friends). It is important to consider all these factors from the outset if you are to treat the individual efficiently. An holistic approach is essential.

Treatment for stroke and TIA should be approached both anatomically and pathologically. The anatomical approach concerns the vascular territory involved and the cerebral structures affected. The pathological approach will consider whether an infarction or a haemorrhage is the cause of the stroke. Determining the cause may be clinically difficult but is important for patient management and prognosis.

1. Epidemiology

Incidence
Prevalence
Case fatality and mortality
Types of stroke
Risk factors for ischaemic stroke
Risk factors for haemorrhagic stroke
Conclusion

Incidence

Stroke incidence, defined as the number of acute strokes per year, depends primarily on the age, sex, and racial mix of the population; whether only first strokes or all strokes are counted; whether transient ischaemic attacks (TIAs) are included as well as completed strokes; and the diagnostic criteria used. There is a global deficiency in accurate and comparable incidence data for stroke. Important incidence studies have come from North America, Europe, Japan and Australasia, but these can be difficult to compare as the studies were not carried out using the same parameters.

The average age-adjusted incidence rate of first strokes has been reported to be 114 per 100,000 of the population but ranges from 81–150 per 100,000 in different studies. Men have 30–80% higher rates than women. The incidence of stroke doubles with every decade after 55 years of age. For example, between 1980 and 1984 in Rochester, MN, USA, stroke incidence increased nearly nine-fold between ages 55 to 64 and 85 years or over. Within a society that is increasingly becoming more aged, there will be an increasing stroke occurrence for two reasons:

- a direct and predictable effect of a growing proportion of elderly individuals within that population

- a disproportionately increased stroke risk among the older age groups.

> Men have a 30–80% higher incidence rate of stroke compared to women

Race may cause variation in stroke incidence rates – rates are 50% higher in African-American men than in Caucasian men, and 130% higher in African-American women than in Caucasian women. A study in London, England found increased incidence of stroke among those in the black ethnic group, older age group, male sex and lower social class. The incidence of stroke in Scotland may actually be higher than defined in population studies from elsewhere in the UK. In the UK, the incidence of all strokes (first and recurrent) is 2.4 per 1000 persons per year. Among people aged 55–64 years the incidence of first stroke is two per 1000 per year; this rises to 20 per 1000 per year in those aged over 85 years. Hospital-based record linkage studies in Scotland suggest that the annual incidence is approximately three per 1000 of the population, however, this may be an underestimation. First-ever strokes account for about 75% of acute events and recurrent strokes account for about 25%. The risk of stroke recurrence is high among survivors – approximately 7% for at least five years after the initial event.

> After a stroke, the risk of stroke recurrence in survivors is 7% for at least five years after the first event

Prevalence

Stroke prevalence – the number of living persons at any given time who have had a stroke – depends on the interaction of incidence and survival. In developed countries the incidence is high. Studies have found stroke prevalence to be:

- 500–800 cases per 100,000 population in Rochester, MN, USA

- 833 per 100,000 in New Zealand
- 1030 per 100,000 men in Finland
- as high as between 1470 and 1750 per 100,000 in the UK.

In Scotland it has been estimated that the prevalence is approximately 1000 per 100,000 of the population. Within the UK it has been estimated that there are 110,000 first strokes and 30,000 recurrent strokes during the course of one year and there are approximately 500,000 stroke survivors. Stroke is clearly a very important disease as shown by Table 1.1 where the incidence and prevalence of common neurological problems are compared with stroke.

> Each year there are approximately 110,000 first strokes and 30,000 recurrent strokes in the UK

Case fatality and mortality

In most Western populations, stroke is the third most common cause of death after ischaemic heart disease and all cancers, accounting for one in 10 of all deaths each year. The importance of stroke as a cause of death in Scotland is shown in Figure 1.1.

There has been a significant decline in stroke mortality in most Western countries and Japan since the 1950s, although there is evidence that this decline in mortality may be levelling off. Women have shown the more dramatic decline in stroke at all ages. The decline

probably reflects the combined effects of better control of modifiable risk factors (such as hypertension), earlier accurate diagnosis and better acute management of the patient. An example of the downward trend in stroke mortality is taken from the study of Shahar et al (Figure 1.2).

In some countries, however, such as those in Eastern Europe, there have been recent increases in stroke mortality.

The average 30-day case fatality rate from stroke in the 1970s and 1980s was 21%, ranging from 17% to 34%; one-year mortality ranged from 25–40%; and three-year mortality ranged from 32–60%. Ten-year stroke survival in the Framingham Study is 35%. Therefore, about half of the people with first strokes live for three or more years and more than one-third live for 10 years. Mortality rates for intracerebral haemorrhages are much higher than those for infarction. In Rochester, MN, USA, the 30-day case fatality rate was 48% for intracerebral haemorrhage compared with 17% for all strokes.

Stroke mortality has declined further in recent years and this may be attributed to a combination of better acute care, reduced stroke severity and earlier and more accurate diagnosis. Approximately 30% of stroke patients die within the first three weeks and for those who survive beyond 30 days, 36% of deaths are due to first or recurrent stroke.

Table 1.1
Comparison of approximate incidence and prevalence of common neurological problems in UK

Disease	Incidence (per million per year)	Prevalence (per million per year)
Completed stroke	2200	36,000
Moderate/severe traumatic brain injury	200	1500
Parkinson's disease	200	720
Multiple sclerosis	40	500
Motor neurone disease	20	60

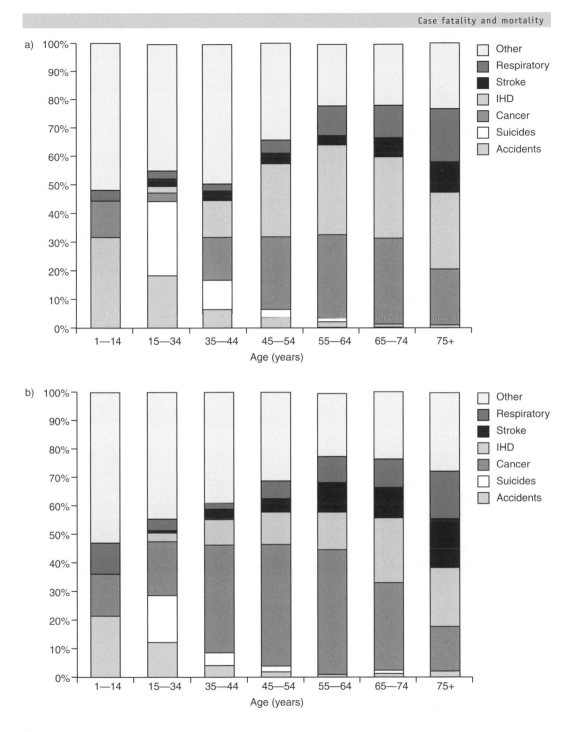

Figure 1.1

Cause of death by age in Scotland in 1997.

a) represents males and b) represents females

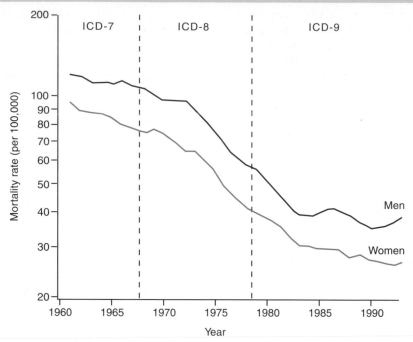

Figure 1.2

Age-adjusted stroke mortality among men and women, aged 30–74: Minneapolis-St Paul, 1960–1994.

Reprinted with permission from Shahar *et al. Stroke* 1997; **28**: 275–9

> Stroke rates have been declining owing to better acute care, reduced stroke severity and more accurate diagnosis

The countries with low stroke mortality rates and those that showed steep declines from a previously high stroke mortality rate during the past 25 years are affluent industrialized countries. Certain countries did particularly well. Japan and Finland, which had, respectively, the highest and the second highest rate of stroke mortality in the world at the beginning of the 1970s, had significant drops. In certain countries, such as Australia and the USA, the decline was remarkable as these countries started from a more favourable position. The decline in stroke mortality has been occurring in both those below and above 75 years of age, indicating a general improvement in the risk of stroke and not just a shift of stroke mortality toward the older age groups. The difference between the trends observed in the two age groups has been attributed to a shift of stroke onset to the latter age group.

The accelerated decline in stroke mortality during the late 1970s and the early 1980s in a number of industrialized countries has been documented in a number of studies – this can, in part, be attributed to improvements in the detection and treatment of hypertension. In the 1970s studies reported the declining trends in both the incidence and case fatality of stroke during that decade. However, more recent studies which are supported by data from their population-based stroke registers have not been able to show any significant decline in the incidence of stroke. Still, mortality from stroke has continued to decline throughout the 1970s and the 1980s in these countries, suggesting that acute stroke events have become milder and that the prevalence of stroke survivors in these communities is increasing. Whether this decline in mortality from stroke can be attributed to an improvement in the control of hypertension has been debated. If reduction in hypertension is responsible, it is more likely that a decrease in the prevalence of some environmental factors (such as decrease in the intake of dietary salt and saturated fat) has contributed more to the decrease in stroke mortality than has pharmacological treatment of hypertension itself. It has even been suggested that a reduction in salt intake by 50 mmol/day in the entire population would be 1.5 times more effective than pharmacological treatment of all hypertensive patients to reduce stroke mortality in the community. Antihypertensive treatment trials are associated with a decrease in the incidence and mortality from stroke.

It is also likely that some risk factors for stroke are increasing and this could cause the decline in mortality to slow down and therefore a possible upturn in stroke incidence. The data available seem to support this hypothesis, insomuch as the incidence of alcohol consumption, abdominal obesity and diabetes is increasing in most countries. In addition, while hypertension may not be increasing in prevalence and control may be improving, the incidence of congestive heart failure seems to be increasing, and it is possible that the prevalence of atrial fibrillation, an important risk factor for stroke, might also be increasing. Both of these are important risk factors for stroke. These trends may be primarily related to the improved long-term survival of patients with hypertension and also those with ischaemic heart disease, who are at very high risk of stroke.

> Congestive heart failure, atrial fibrillation and hypertension are important risk factors for stroke

Mortality can be divided into short-term case fatality and long-term mortality. There is evidence that both have been declining. Twenty-eight day case fatality from stroke has been declining. The case fatality in milder strokes and in the most severe strokes who are too ill to be hospitalized cannot be determined accurately, but in certain studies the effect of this can be minimized. In part this is due to stroke survival in hospital which has been shown to be improving. An example of this is a study in older patients from Portland, OR, USA. The improvement in survival curves is illustrated in Figure 1.3, the survival gain in the short term is translated into a long-term gain.

The odds ratio (OR) of dying within 28 days improved 0.55 (95% confidence interval (CI) 0.39–0.77) from the 1970 level to the 1985 level in Minnesota. The age- and sex-adjusted five-year survival of definite stroke also improved significantly from 1970 to 1985 (OR 0.72; 95% CI 0.54–0.96) in that study. Survival in hospital is better in well organized stroke units. Factors that tend to improve survival include a shorter time to start of mobilization and therapy training, increased use of oxygen, heparin, intravenous saline solutions and antipyretics, and attention to blood pressure control. Other factors that may be equally or more important include the effects of characteristic features of a stroke unit such as a specially trained staff, teamwork and involvement of relatives in a co-ordinated care package.

Long-term survival

The long-term survival among stroke patients is poorer than an age- and sex-matched sample from the same community. An example of this is illustrated in the Kaplan-Meier survival plot from a study in Perth, Western Australia (Figure 1.4).

> Stroke rates increase with age although the actual stroke can occur at any time of life

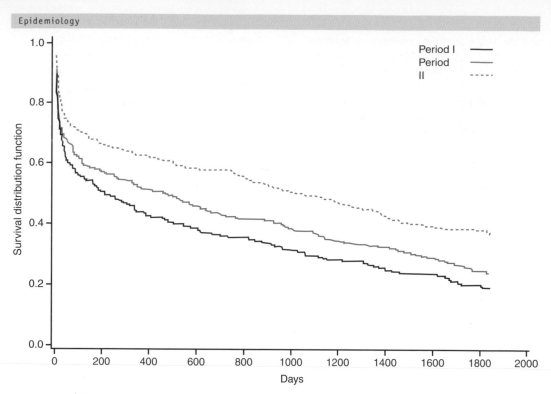

Figure 1.3

Five-year period-specific survival curves following acute hospitalized strokes in patients 65 years and older in each period, using Kaplan-Meier estimates. Period 1 indicates 1967–1971; period 2 1974–1978; and period 3 1981–1985.

Adapted from Barker WH, Mullooly JP. *Stroke* 1997; **28**: 284–90

Types of stroke

A person of any age may be affected by stroke, although it becomes more common with increasing age. The spectrum of illness can range from a minor episode (a transient ischaemic attack, or TIA) lasting a few minutes or hours, to a major life threatening or disabling event.

The aetiologies of stroke can be classified broadly into:

- atherothrombotic brain infarction
- haemorrhage
- other causes.

Haemorrhages may be intracerebral or subarachnoid. Subdural haematomas can present

in a similar way but are generally classified separately. Accurate diagnoses are difficult to achieve based on clinical impressions alone and require information from laboratory studies including computerized tomography (CT) scanning, magnetic resonance imaging (MRI) and magnetic resonance angiography. Even with laboratory studies, however, the diagnosis represents a 'best clinical guess' in a substantial number of patients. Definitions differ among studies and need to be taken into account when interpreting the results.

Accurate diagnosis requires imaging techniques

Stroke is not a homogeneous condition. There are clear pathological sub-types – cerebral

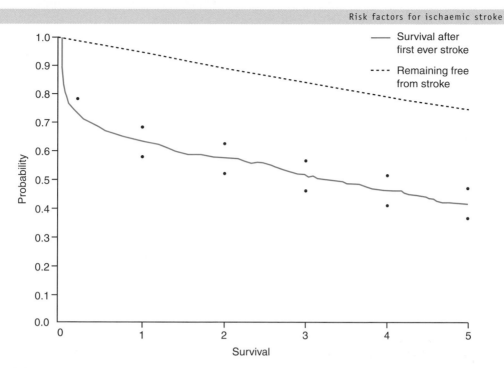

Figure 1.4
Kaplan-Meier curve showing the probability of survival after a first-ever stroke (solid line), compared with the expected probability in the same general population remaining free from a first stroke (dotted line), derived from Perth Community Stroke Study incidence data 1989–1990. Dots on either side of the solid line indicate 95% confidence intervals.

infarction, primary intra-cerebral haemorrhage and sub-arachnoid haemorrhage – with over 100 potential underlying causes. Keeping in mind uncertainties about diagnostic accuracy, community-based studies report that 61–81% of first strokes represent infarctions, 8–16% intracerebral haemorrhages, and 4–8% subarachnoid haemorrhages An accurate diagnosis is important because of the relationship of aetiology to mortality, recurrence rates, and choice of treatment.

In the UK, over 80% of first strokes are due to cerebral infarction, about 10% result from primary intracerebral haemorrhage and approximately 5% are due to sub-arachnoid haemorrhage.

The Oxfordshire Community Stroke Project (OCSP) devised simple criteria for sub-dividing strokes on clinical and investigational grounds to make presumptions about pathology. The OCSP divided strokes in to total anterior circulation strokes, partial anterior circulation strokes, lacunar strokes and posterior circulation strokes. Another useful pathological classification scheme for brain infarction (ischaemic strokes) developed in the multicentre Trial of Org 10172 in Acute Stroke Treatment (TOAST) in the USA is said to have the advantages of clinical relevance and reliability. This system divides infarctions into large artery atherosclerosis, cardioembolism, small vessel occlusions or infarcts of undetermined cause.

Risk factors for ischaemic stroke

In most cases, strokes are not simply caused by one factor. They tend to occur because multiple risk factors are present in susceptible individuals. Most of the burden of stroke is due to ischaemic stroke and the risk factors for these have been studied extensively. Some of the risk factors are shared with haemorrhagic causes of stroke, but some are not.

Risk factors for ischaemic stroke can be divided into those that are potentially modifiable and those that are not. A list of important risk factors for stroke is shown in Table 1.2. Most important among modifiable risk factors are:

- TIAs
- hypertension
- diabetes mellitus
- atrial fibrillation
- left ventricular hypertrophy
- cigarette smoking.

Prior stroke, age, sex, race and family history are important non-modifiable factors. Stroke is more often associated with one or more risk factors

Table 1.2
Recognized risk factors for ischaemic stroke

Well-documented risk factors	Less well-documented risk factors
Non-modifiable	***Potentially modifiable***
age	elevated blood cholesterol and lipids
gender	cardiac disease
hereditary/familial factors	cardiomyopathy
race/ethnicity	segmental wall motion abnormalities
geographic location	nonbacterial endocarditis
	mitral annular calcification
Modifiable, value established	mitral valve prolapse
hypertension	valve strands
cardiac disease	spontaneous echocardiographic contrast
atrial fibrillation	aortic stenosis
infective endocarditis	patent foramen ovale
mitral stenosis	atrial septal aneurysm
recent large myocardial infarction	use of oral contraceptives
cigarette smoking	consumption of alcohol
sickle cell disease	use of illicit drugs
transient ischaemic attacks	physical inactivity
asymptomatic carotid stenosis	obesity
diabetes mellitus	elevated haematocrit
hyperhomocysteinaemia	dietary factors
left ventricular hypertrophy	hyperinsulinaemia and insulin resistance
	acute triggers (stress)
	migraine
	hypercoagulability and inflammation
	fibrin formation and fibrinolysis
	fibrinogen
	anticardiolipin antibodies
	genetic and acquired causes
	subclinical diseases
	intimal-medial thickness
	aortic atheroma
	ankle:brachial blood pressure ratio
	infarct-like lesions on MRI
	socioeconomic features
	infections
	Non-modifiable
	season and climate

MRI, magnetic resonance imaging

and these risk factors appear to have a greater than additive effect. Risk factors for different subtypes of ischaemic stroke are similar.

> The risk of stroke increases with rising blood pressure. When blood pressure is above 160/90 mmHg, the risk of stroke becomes very high

Age

Advancing age is an important risk factor for stroke. It is unmodifiable but confers a relative risk itself of approximately 2.2 per decade increase. (Many of the studies did not study those over 75 years of age.) The importance of certain risk factors appears to reduce with increasing age, for example hypertension. The relative risk of stroke if one had an increased diastolic blood pressure was two for those over 65 years, compared to five for those aged 45–64 and 10 for those under 45 years. In the Framingham study as age increases progressively from 50 to 80 years, so the relative risks associated with hypertension, ischaemic heart disease, heart failure and atrial fibrillation (AF) all decrease. The relative risks associated with diabetes and smoking also decrease with age. Although the relative risk diminishes with age, the attributable risk is maintained or rises.

Hypertension

The paramount potentially modifiable risk factor for stroke is hypertension. The relationship is with both diastolic and systolic blood pressure and is especially strong for levels above 160/95 mmHg. The continuing rise in risk with systolic and diastolic blood pressure is seen in studies of primary stroke and secondary stroke. All measures of blood pressure, including systolic, diastolic, and pulse pressure, are associated with the incidence of stroke. The frequency of hypertension as a risk factor has been found to be similar among patients with stroke due to large-vessel disease, cardioembolic stroke and lacunae. Hypertension was the most frequent end-point in at least 10 major hypertension treatment studies, and this demonstrates that hypertension is intimately linked to stroke. Treatment of stroke patients with an antihypertensive regime has been shown to be beneficial.

Cardiac disease

The presence of cardiac abnormalities, such as AF, left ventricular hypertrophy, coronary heart disease and congestive heart failure, increases the risk of stroke at any blood pressure. Acute myocardial infarction and atrial fibrillation predispose to embolism from cardiac thrombi and nearly 15% of strokes in the Framingham Study have been attributed to atrial fibrillation. The risk of cerebral infarction is five times higher in individuals with electrocardiographic evidence of left ventricular hypertrophy even after other risk factors are taken into account. Patent foramen ovale are increasingly being recognized as a potential cause of stroke.

Atrial fibrillation

Atrial fibrillation increases in prevalence with age; 5% of people aged over 65 years have AF. Atrial fibrillation confers a five-fold increased risk of stroke. The risk of stroke varies with age, hypertension, previous stroke or previous TIA. The effects of these factors are illustrated in Table 1.3.

Table 1.3
Risk of stroke among patients with atrial fibrillation

Age	Risk factors present	Annual risk of stroke (%)
<65 years	None	1.0
	One or more	4.9
65–75 years	None	4.3
	One or more	5.7
>75 years	None	3.5
	One or more	8.1

Risk factors = hypertension, previous stroke, previous TIA

In the Stroke Prevention in Atrial Fibrillation (SPAF) study, recent heart failure, hypertension and previous thrombo-embolism were identified as additional risks, with the risk of stroke increasing from 2.5% per year with no factor present to 7.2% per year with one factor present and 17.6% per year with two or three factors present. Echocardiographic findings, including left ventricular dysfunction and atrial size over 4.7 cm, added additional risk to the clinical findings of SPAF. The risk was 1% per year for no factors, 6% per year for two factors and 18.6% per year for three or more of those factors.

Warfarin as a long-term secondary prevention therapy is not recommended for ischaemic stroke patients who are in sinus rhythm. The Stroke Prevention in Reversible Ischemia Trial (SPIRIT) comparing aspirin with warfarin (international normalized ratio [INR] target range 3.0–4.5) was stopped early because of an excess of cerebral haemorrhage in the anticoagulated group. A further study comparing warfarin (INR target range 1.4–2.8) with antiplatelet therapy did not show advantages for warfarin over aspirin.

Recently it has been established that patients with AF are more likely than controls to have aortic atheromatous plaques, which themselves can be a potent risk factor for stroke, and patients with atrial fibrillation tend to be elderly and may have a worse overall cardiovascular risk profile than younger patients and patients without AF. For those with intermittent AF the risk of subsequent stroke appears as high as it is for those with established atrial fibrillation.

Antiplatelet therapy in relation to atherosclerosis

Antiplatelet agents play an important role in preventing ischaemic stroke and TIA in those at risk. A diagrammatic representation of their role is shown in Figure 1.5.

For patients with ischaemic stroke in sinus rhythm, aspirin has a modest effect in reducing death and disability after an acute episode. Aspirin is the most commonly used antiplatelet drug. Aspirin is a cyclo-oxygenase inhibitor that irreversibly acetylates the enzyme cyclo-oxygenase.

Lipids

The relationship between blood lipids and stroke is not clear even though increased lipid levels have been related to carotid artery disease. Epidemiological studies of the relationship between cholesterol and stroke have been confusing. The Prospective Studies Collaboration

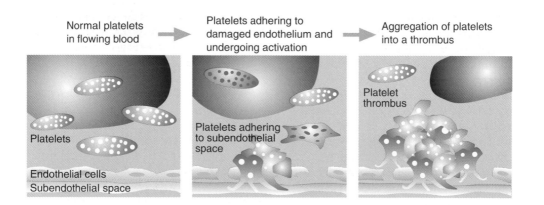

Figure 1.5
How platelets adhere to damaged endothelium, are activated and then aggregate into a thrombus

found no link between cholesterol concentration and stroke. Low serum cholesterol has been found in Hawaiian, Japanese and other populations despite an increased incidence of stroke, but the underlying pathology is usually cerebral haemorrhage. Some have suggested that an association between stroke and cholesterol may exist at both extremes of cholesterol distribution, but of course low cholesterol can be associated with a number of serious co-morbid conditions. Treatment of hypercholesterolaemia in stroke patients is not certainly recommended at present in the presence of ischaemic heart disease (IHD). The Heart Protection Study (HPS) suggests there is a benefit.

Meta-analyses of trials of HMGCoA reductase inhibitor (statin) therapy both in primary and secondary prevention of IHD have shown there were substantial reductions in the incidence of stroke as well as myocardial disease among those receiving active therapy. Whether lowering cholesterol with statin drugs among stroke patients who have no evidence of cardiac disease will result in reduction of end-points is currently being tested in the Stroke Prevention by Aggressive Reduction in Cholesterol Level (SPARCL) trial.

Diabetes mellitus

Diabetes mellitus is a serious risk factor for stroke, conferring an up to three-fold increased risk of stroke. In the United Kingdom Prospective Diabetes Study (UKPDS) 33 type II diabetics receiving intensive therapy with sulphonylureas or insulin to improve blood glucose control experienced a reduction of microvascular complications but not macrovascular disease. In the UKPDS 34, type II diabetics who were overweight showed intensive blood glucose control with metformin compared to other hypoglycaemic drugs with similar intensive control reduced stroke, myocardial infarction and death by 5–10%.

> Patients with diabetes have their risk of stroke increased three-fold

Smoking

The association of cigarette smoking with stroke holds for thrombotic strokes, as well as intracerebral and subarachnoid haemorrhages. Cigarette smoking, long established as a risk factor for coronary artery disease, has more recently been found to be an independent determinant of stroke. In case-control and cohort studies, the effect of cigarette smoking remained significant after adjustment for other factors and a dose–response relationship was apparent. A meta-analysis of 32 studies found that smoking increased the risk of stroke by about 50% in both sexes and all age groups, and that risk was directly related to the number of cigarettes smoked per day. For people with coronary heart disease, even passive smoking is dangerous and even short exposure can affect endothelial function in the circulation. It is likely that the cerebral circulation will also be affected.

Smoking causes endothelial dysfunction and activates platelets. This probably has a synergistic adverse effect. Animal models have shown that exposure to small amounts of cigarette smoke promotes the development of atherosclerotic plaques. Endothelial dysfunction may be at the heart of the development of atherosclerosis. Normal endothelial cells promote vasodilatation and inhibit atherosclerosis and thrombosis, in part because of the release of nitric oxide. Dysfunctional endothelial cells, on the other hand, contribute to vasoconstriction, atherogenesis and thrombosis. Cardiovascular risk factors contribute individually to endothelial dysfunction and appear to be additive. One possible unifying hypothesis for the effects of risk factors is that they increase the oxidative stress that mediates these effects. Thus, reduction of risk factors improves endothelial function and reduces clinical cardiovascular events. For example, in patients with dyslipidaemia, lipid lowering appears to improve endothelial function both acutely and chronically. The central role of atherosclerosis is shown in Figure 1.6.

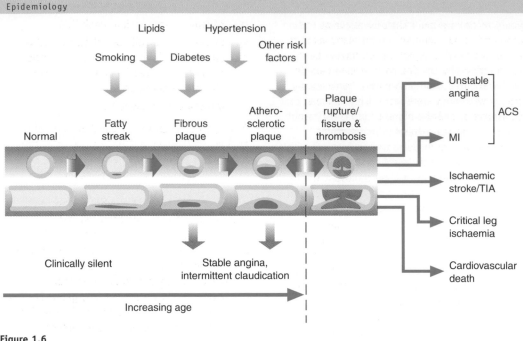

Figure 1.6
Atherosclerosis – risk factors and effects.

ACS, acute coronary syndrome; TIA, transient ischaemic attack, MI, myocardial infarction

The risk of stroke falls quickly when smoking ceases, falling to the level of non-smokers within five years of quitting. Brief advice from medical practitioners alone only increases the cessation rate by 2.5%. However, more intensive cessation support and counselling further improve cessation rates. Nicotine replacement therapy can double quitting rates and the use of this or the newer drug, bupropion, together with counselling, can increase the success rate of quitting smoking.

Alcohol

The role of alcohol as a risk factor is more controversial. Regular moderate alcohol intake may be protective against stroke. Regular excessive intake might predispose to haemorrhage as platelet aggregation, leukocyte aggregation and adhesion are diminished. Clotting factor production may be reduced with excessive consumption. Heavy binge drinking may be particularly problematic. In this situation, alcohol may increase the risk for

stroke through various mechanisms that include:

- hypertension
- hypercoaguable states
- cardiac arrhythmia
- cerebral blood flow reductions associated with the withdrawal phase.

> Binge drinking can increase stroke risk by causing hypertension, hypercoagulable states, cardiac arrhythmia and reduction in cerebral blood flow

Consumption of three or more drinks of alcohol per day approximately doubles the risk of hypertension. The actual contribution of alcohol to the prevalence of hypertension in a population varies according to the prevalence of heavy drinking and the prevalence of hypertension in that population. Alcohol has been estimated to account for about 5–20% of hypertension in populations. Excessive alcohol consumption has been known for many years to be associated with hypertension, having been first described by the French physician Camille Lian, who noted that sailors who drank several litres of wine daily were more likely to have hypertension, and the blood pressure (BP) went up with increasing alcohol intake. Decrease in alcohol consumption is associated with reduction in blood pressure. This effect is also seen among alcoholics. Within several days of abstention the hypertensive effect of alcohol usually subsides. The relationship between alcohol intake and BP is strongest for alcohol drunk within the previous 24 hours. Drinkers who concentrate their drinking at weekends will find they have significantly higher blood pressure on Mondays than on Thursdays – this effect is not seen in those who drink daily. Although some studies suggest that one type of alcoholic beverage, such as beer or liquor, is more strongly associated with BP levels than another, it appears that the relationship between alcohol and BP levels is more dependent on the actual amount of alcohol ingested. Alcohol intake can be associated with resistance to antihypertensive medication therapy; poor compliance may be a factor, although interference with the blood pressure lowering effects of some drugs probably occurs. Randomized controlled trials have examined the relationship between reduction in alcohol consumption and BP. Although some studies have been small they lend support to the epidemiological relationship of alcohol and BP.

The hypertensive effect of alcohol is thought to stem from a chronic state of alcohol withdrawal in frequent, heavy drinkers, but there is much evidence in favour of a direct effect of alcohol on BP. Suggested mediators of a direct effect include:

- stimulation of the sympathetic nervous system, endothelin, renin–angiotensin–aldosterone system, insulin (or insulin resistance) or cortisol
- inhibition of vascular relaxing substances, eg nitric oxide

- calcium or magnesium depletion
- increased intracellular calcium or other electrolytes in vascular smooth muscle, possibly mediated by changes in membrane electrolyte transport
- increased acetaldehyde.

Of the different proposed mechanisms, there appears to be more evidence to support the role of the sympathetic nervous system, or cellular transport and electrolytes, or both.

Higher intake levels of alcohol are not only associated with an increased risk for hypertension. Other complications of high alcohol intake will alter the risk for stroke, eg cardiomyopathy and other cardiac complications, certain kinds of cancer, hepatitis, cirrhosis, pancreatitis, gastritis, and other effects of alcohol abuse and dependence, including suicide, accidents and violence.

Elimination of heavy drinking and binge drinking is probably sensible. Excessive consumption of alcohol is sometimes associated with obesity and obesity itself has also been linked to an increased incidence of stroke. However, there is also evidence that light to moderate drinking can reduce the risk for stroke and that drinking wine may be preferable to consumption of other types of alcohol.

Beneficial effects of alcohol ingestion are also well known. Low to moderate alcohol intake is associated with a lower incidence of atherosclerotic cardiovascular events, such as myocardial infarction (MI) and atherothrombotic stroke, compared with no alcohol ingestion. The explanation for these epidemiologically observed benefits of alcohol may be related to increases in high-density lipoprotein (HDL) and apolipoproteins A_1 and A_2, antioxidant effects and reduced platelet aggregability.

Obviously, alcohol consumption has both beneficial and detrimental effects, and therefore it would seem that heavy drinking and binge drinking may be the main risk factor for stroke.

Prior stroke or TIA

People who have suffered previous stroke or TIA are at a high risk of further strokes – approximately 10% in the first year and 5% per year thereafter. The risk of recurrent stroke is highest in the first six months after stroke.

> The risk of having a recurrent stroke is highest in the six months following the first stroke or TIA

The risk of recurrence after minor stroke and TIA is high. Among the 184 people with a TIA in the Oxfordshire Community Stroke Project the risk of stroke was 4.4% in the first month (relative risk [RR] = 80), 8.8% in the first six months and 11.6% in the first year after the event (RR = 13). The risk of stroke was 5.9% per year over five years (RR = 7), risk of death was 6.3% per year and the combined risk of MI, stroke or vascular death was 8.4% per year. The TIA predicted the vascular territory of the forthcoming stroke in only 60% of cases.

Outcome after TIA depends on how the patients were selected for study. In hospital-referred patients the risk was 6.6% in the first year and 3.4% per year over five years. Among a study of 469 patients with TIAs, important risk factors for subsequent stroke included:

- age
- gender
- number of TIAs in the preceding three months
- peripheral arterial disease
- left ventricular hypertrophy
- residual neurological findings
- having both vertebral and carotid territory TIAs
- amaurosis fugax.

Prognostic models have been developed, but in clinical practice they are of limited utility because, unfortunately, the majority of strokes do seem to occur in those without adverse prognostic features. The risk for subsequent MI is high among TIA patients, so an overall cardiovascular risk reduction strategy is recommended.

> TIAs do not always predict the vascular territory that will be affected by a forthcoming stroke – only 60% of TIAs are predictive

Carotid artery disease

Severe carotid artery stenosis is known to be a strong predictor of subsequent stroke among those presenting with TIA or minor stroke. In asymptomatic patients the risk is low (approximately 1–2% per year). There is a higher risk of silent stroke occurring on the affected side. Carotid artery atherosclerosis is more common when there are two or more other risk factors present, or the patient also has ischaemic heart disease or peripheral arterial disease.

Hyperhomocysteinaemia

> Risk of stroke and cerebrovascular disease are increased as plasma homocysteine levels go up

Hyperhomocysteinaemia has been identified as a risk factor for stroke and cerebrovascular disease in several studies. In a meta-analysis of eight cross-sectional and four longitudinal studies, the overall weighted odds-ratio for disease with a concentration of homocysteine in plasma or serum above the 95-percentile was 3.97 (95% CI 3.07–5.12). This suggests there is a case for a strong relationship between hyperhomocysteinaemia and cerebrovascular disease. The vascular risk appears to rise continuously across the spectrum of elevated plasma homocysteine concentrations. It is at least as important as cholesterol, lipoprotein abnormalities and hypertension and should be part of risk assessment, especially for those at high risk. Moderately elevated plasma homocysteine concentration is readily correctable by folic acid, betaine or vitamin B_{12}

supplementation. It seems logical to assume that a reduction in homocysteine concentration will reduce the risk of ischaemic stroke, but there are as yet no published data to prove this. Indeed, it remains to be determined whether lowering total homocysteine prevents hard clinical outcome events, such as stroke and other serious vascular events. An alternative explanation for the observed association between elevated total homocysteine and stroke is a confounding effect of other factors associated with hyperhomocysteinaemia (eg an atherogenic diet, cysteine deficiency, folate deficiency, cigarette smoking and renal impairment) or perhaps even the acute vascular events themselves, where tissue damage might temporarily increase total homocysteine levels.

Other risk factors

Certain risk factors for stroke and the relative risk attributed to these risk factors are tabulated in Table 1.4. In addition, some of the risk factors for stroke and their relationship to stroke risk are shown in Figure 1.7. Potential risk factors attracting increased interest include inflammatory processes and infectious agents.

Risk factors for haemorrhagic stroke

While many risk factors are shared between cerebral infarction and cerebral haemorrhage, risk factors for primary parenchymal intracranial haemorrhage (Table 1.5) are slightly different from those for cerebral infarction. Of particular relevance are age, male gender, race, hypertension, heavy use of alcohol, anticoagulant use and amyloid angiopathy. The latter may be particularly common with increasing age and should be suspected when other risk factors for haemorrhagic stroke have been excluded. Although intervention trials for haemorrhagic stroke are not common, the Perindopril Protection Against Recurrent Stroke Study (PROGRESS) has shown that blood pressure reduction in patients with cerebral haemorrhage results in reduction of further stroke and vascular end-points.

Table 1.4
Risk factors for stroke and their associated relative risk

Stroke risk factor	RR*
Inherent factors	
advancing age (per decade)	2.2
race	<2
Genetic factors	
family history	1.4–2
monozygotic twins	1–5
homocysteinaemia	5–7
(highest versus lowest quartile)	
monozygotic twins	1–5
Physiological factors	
blood pressure	2.3
forced expiratory volume	2
cholesterol	NA
lipoprotein	NA
fibrinogen (highest versus lowest quartile)	2.5
haematocrit	NA
endogenous tPA (top 5% versus rest)	3.5
obesity	1–2
diabetes mellitus	2–3
snoring	2
Behaviours	
alcohol excess (>30 units/week)	2.5–4
smoking	2
dietary vitamin C (top versus bottom third)	2
dietary potassium (lowest third versus rest)	2–5
exercise	0.3–0.5
life events	2
hormone replacement therapy	0.5–2
combined oral contraceptive	2.5–3
Environmental factors	
ambient temperature	NA
air pollution	NA
Social characteristics	
social class	1.6–3.5
Comorbidity factors	
heart failure	2.5–4.4
ischaemic heart disease	2.5
atrial fibrillation	5
carotid bruit	2–3
carotid occlusion (complete)	NA
carotid occlusion (partial)	NA
aortic arch atheroma	5
peripheral occlusive arterial disease	NA
TIA	7

continued

Table 1.4 – *continued*

Stroke risk factor	RR*
Comorbidity factors – *continued*	
previous stroke	9–15
acute infections	5
warfarin treatment	7–10
migraine	1.3–1.8
Other factors	
birth weight (per 454g increase)	0.9
post-partum	8.7

*RR = relative risk *quoted from original papers or Ebrahim and Harwood*; NA = not available, tPA = tissue plasminogen

Table 1.5
Risk factors for haemorrhagic stroke

- Hypertension
- Amyloid angiopathy
- AV malformation
- Intracranial aneurysm
- Coagulopathy
- Vasculitis
- Alcohol abuse
- Cocaine abuse
- Haemorrhagic transformation of infarct
- Cavernous angioma
- Venous angioma
- Dural venous sinus thrombosis
- Intracranial neoplasm

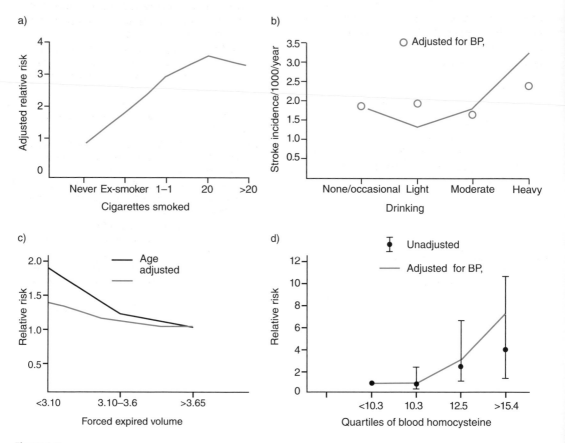

Figure 1.7
Relationship between certain risk factors for stroke and stroke risk. From the British Regional Heart Study.

BP, blood pressure

Reprinted from Shaper AG *et al. BMJ* 1991; **302**: 1111–15 with permission from the BMJ publishing group; reprinted with permission from Elsevier, Perry IJ *et al. Lancet* 1996; **346**: 1395–8

Conclusion

The most important modifiable risk factors for stroke therefore include hypertension, cigarette smoking, AF, left ventricular hypertrophy and TIAs, and it is hoped that in the future, better, more targeted primary prevention will help reduce the burden of stroke in the community. Such strategies have recently been reviewed by consensus. By targeting six important stroke risk factors (hypertension, MI, atrial fibrillation, diabetes mellitus, blood lipids and asymptomatic carotid artery stenosis) and four lifestyle factors (cigarette smoking, alcohol use, physical activity and diet), it has been suggested that the incidence of first stroke can be reduced. One important component in preventing first stroke is improving patient adherence to changes in lifestyle and to medication regimes.

> Incidence of first stroke may be reduced by altering 10 modifiable risk factors: cigarette smoking, alcohol consumption, physical inactivity, diet, hypertension, MI, AF, diabetes, blood lipid levels and asymptomatic carotid artery stenosis

Further reading

Bamford J, Sandercock P, Dennis M et al. A prospective study of acute cerebrovascular disease in the community: the Oxfordshire Community Stroke Project – 1981–86. 2. Incidence, case fatality rates and overall outcome at one year of cerebral infarction, primary intracerebral and subarachnoid haemorrhage. J Neurol Neurosurg Psychiatry 1990; 53: 16–22.

Bonita R, Solomon N, Broad JB. Prevalence of stroke and stroke-related disability. Estimates from the Auckland stroke studies. Stroke 1997; 28: 1898–1902.

Bonita R, Stewart A, Beaglehole R. International trends in stroke mortality: 1970–1985. Stroke 1990; 21: 989–92.

Dennis MS, Burn JP, Sandercock PA et al. Long-term survival after first-ever stroke: the Oxfordshire Community Stroke Project. Stroke 1993; 24: 796–800.

Gorelick PB, Sacco RL, Smith DB et al. Prevention of a first stroke: a review of guidelines and a multidisciplinary consensus statement from the National Stroke Association. JAMA 1999; 281: 1112–20.

Hankey GJ, Jamrozik K, Broadhurst RJ et al. Five-year survival after first-ever stroke and related prognostic factors in the Perth Community Stroke Study. Stroke 2000; 31: 2080–6.

Indredavik B, Bakke F, Slordahl SA et al. Treatment in a combined acute and rehabilitation stroke unit: which aspects are most important? Stroke 1999; 30: 917–23.

Lian C. L'alcoholisme cause d'hypertension artérielle. Bull Acad Med (Paris) 1915; 74: 525–8.

MacMahon S, Rodgers A. The epidemiological association between blood pressure and stroke: implications for primary and secondary prevention. Hypertens Res 1994; 17: S23–S32.

MacWalter RS, Ersoy Y, Wolfson DR. Cerebral Haemorrhage. Parenchymal intracranial haemorrhage. Gerontology 2001; 47: 119–30.

Murray CJ, Lopez AD. Global mortality, disability, and the contribution of risk factors: Global Burden of Disease Study. Lancet 1997; 349: 1436–42.

O'Mahony PG, Thomson RG, Dobson R et al. The prevalence of stroke and associated disability. J Publ Health Med 1999; 21: 166–71.

Shinton R, Beevers G. Meta-analysis of relation between cigarette smoking and stroke. BMJ 1989; 298: 789–94.

Shinton R, Sagar G, Beevers G. The relation of alcohol consumption to cardiovascular risk factors and stroke. The west Birmingham stroke project. J Neurol Neurosurg Psychiatry 1993; 56: 458–62.

Wade DT. Epidemiology of disabling neurological disease: how and why does disability occur? J Neurol Neurosurg Psychiatry 1996; 61: 242–9.

2. Pathophysiology

Atherosclerosis
Cardiac embolism
Lipohyalinosis
Other causes

Atherosclerosis

Atherosclerosis is a complex problem. Atherosclerosis, which comes from the Greek words 'athero' (meaning gruel or paste) and 'sclerosis' (meaning hardness), specifically involves changes to the intimal layer of arteries. It is characterized by a progressive build-up of plaque within the arterial wall and a loss of elasticity.

The artery wall consists of three layers:

- an outer layer of connective tissue
- a second layer of smooth muscle cells and elastic connective tissue
- a third inner layer of endothelial cells.

These cells are aligned with the blood stream and must maintain a non-stick inner surface to avoid turbulence that can lead to thrombotic and coagulant activities.

Any mechanical or chemical injury can damage the endothelial cell monolayer or the non-stick surface of endothelial cells. This alters the normal laminar blood flow and provides sites for further thrombocyte adhesion and aggregation, leading to the formation of thrombi in the arterial wall. Alterations of the endothelium cause monocytes (white blood cells) to stick to the previously non-stick endothelial layer and the intima itself, where they become active macrophages. Once macrophages make their way into the intima

they begin scavenging modified low-density lipoprotein (LDL) cholesterol. This modified LDL cholesterol results in substantial cholesterol accumulation and foam cell formation in macrophages. The most relevant modification of LDL that appears to occur is oxidation by free-radicals or certain enzymes. These lesions, called fibrous plaques, are adjacent to the arterial lining and increase in size, thus narrowing the arterial lumen. Fibrous plaques are soon covered by a thick dome of connective tissue with embedded smooth muscle cells that usually overlay a core of lipid and necrotic debris.

With time the plaques become calcified and may undergo further changes leading to a partial reduction or total block of blood flow through an artery. If blood is unable to flow through the vessels, it cannot nourish the tissues or remove harmful waste products.

> Atheromatous plaques build up over time and eventually lead to a partial or complete block of blood flow through an artery

The development of atherosclerosis starts at an early age and continues throughout life. In unfortunate individuals it progresses remarkably rapidly but generally it progresses at a variable rate. Factors that affect the development of atherosclerosis include blood lipid levels, hypertension and diabetes mellitus, and these can be modified. Other factors that are potentially modifiable are inflammatory influences within the plaque and fibrous tissue formation in the plaque. As the plaque continues to expand it may lead directly to thrombotic occlusion. However, the most dangerous situation is the complicated atherosclerotic plaque that can rupture, spilling its fatty and non-fatty contents, which are highly thrombogenic and may cause local thrombosis and occlusion and/or embolism (red embolism with high platelet and leukocyte content), see Figure 2.1.

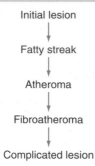

Initial lesion

↓

Fatty streak

↓

Atheroma

↓

Fibroatheroma

↓

Complicated lesion

Figure 2.1
Progression from initial to complicated lesion.

> Rupture of a plaque can lead to an acute thrombus forming with the potential for downstream embolization

Atherosclerotic plaques relevant to stroke can occur at any point between the heart and the brain in the large and medium sized arteries. Most work has focussed on the carotid arteries. Older notions that areas of high shear stress were associated with atherosclerotic plaques have been challenged. The current view is that these plaques occur most commonly in areas of low and oscillating shear stress.

> If atherosclerotic plaques form in a large or medium sized artery between the heart and the brain, they can lead to a stroke

In the Trial of Org 10172 in Acute Stroke Treatment (TOAST) classification large artery atherosclerotic strokes are deemed to occur when patients have clinical and brain imaging findings of either significant (>50%) stenosis or occlusion of a major brain artery or branch cortical artery, presumably due to atherosclerosis.

Clinical findings include those of cerebral cortical impairment (eg aphasia, neglect, restricted motor involvement, etc.) or brain

stem or cerebellar dysfunction depending on which large artery is affected. A history of intermittent claudication, transient ischaemic attacks (TIAs) in the same vascular territory, a carotid bruit, or diminished pulse helps support the clinical diagnosis.

Cortical or cerebellar lesions and brain stem or subcortical hemispheric infarcts greater than 1.5 cm in diameter on computerized tomography or magnetic resonance imaging are considered to be of potential large-artery atherosclerotic origin. Supportive evidence by duplex imaging or arteriography of a stenosis of greater than 50% of an appropriate intracranial or extracranial artery is needed.

Diagnostic studies should exclude potential sources of cardiogenic embolism. The diagnosis of stroke secondary to large-artery atherosclerosis cannot be made if duplex or arteriographic studies are normal or show only minimal changes.

Cardiac embolism

Emboli with a relatively high fibrin content may originate in the heart. Cardiac embolism most commonly complicates acute myocardial infarction and atrial fibrillation (sustained or paroxysmal) although there are rarer situations as shown in Table 2.1. The TOAST classification defines high- and medium-risk situations

> Cardiac embolism complicates atrial fibrillation and myocardial infarction; such embolisms tend to have a high fibrin content

Lipohyalinosis

As well as microatheromatous plaques, which can be responsible for some lacunar infarcts, lipohyalinosis is associated with these infarcts. Lipohyalinosis of small vessels within the brain is associated with lacunar infarcts and is more common among those with hypertension and diabetes mellitus. The TOAST classification defines small-artery occlusion infarcts and this

Table 2.1
TOAST classification of high- and medium-risk sources of cardioembolism

High-risk sources	Medium-risk sources
Mechanical prosthetic valve	Mitral valve prolapse
Mitral stenosis with atrial fibrillation	Mitral valve annulus calcification
Atrial fibrillation (other than lone atrial fibrillation)	Mitral stenosis without atrial fibrillation
Left atrial/atrial appendage thrombus	Left atrial turbulence (smoke)
Sick sinus syndrome	Atrial septal aneurysm
Recent myocardial infarction (<4 weeks)	Patent foramen ovale
Left ventricular thrombus	Atrial flutter
Dilated cardiomyopathy	Lone atrial fibrillation
Akinetic left ventricular segment	Bioprosthetic cardiac valve
Atrial myxoma	Nonbacterial thrombotic endocarditis
Infective endocarditis	Congestive heart failure
	Hypokinetic left ventricular segment
	Myocardial infarction (>4 weeks, <6 months)

includes patients whose strokes are often labelled as lacunar infarcts in other classifications. The patient should have one of the traditional clinical lacunar syndromes and should not have evidence of cerebral cortical dysfunction. There is often a history of diabetes mellitus or hypertension and these support the clinical diagnosis. The computerized tomography scan or magnetic resonance imaging findings are normal, or a relevant brain stem or subcortical hemispheric lesion with a diameter of less than 1.5 cm is demonstrated.

To fit the TOAST criteria, potential cardiac sources for embolism should be absent and evaluation of the large extracranial arteries should not demonstrate a stenosis of greater than 50% in an ipsilateral artery.

Other causes

Cerebral infarction can occur more readily when a hypercoagulable state exists. This can happen in certain circumstances with inherited thrombophilias and in certain inflammatory conditions. These include the antiphospholipid antibody syndrome and other conditions, eg the presence of lupus anticoagulant. Cerebral infarction can also occur in the non-atherosclerotic vasculopathies. Cerebral

infarction can occur with migraine. In younger patients other causes should be actively sought. In states where there is a loss of blood pressure and therefore of brain perfusion, border zone infarction between different arterial territories can occur.

Further reading

Adams HP Jr., Bendixen BH, Kappelle LJ et al. Classification of subtype of acute ischemic stroke. Definitions for use in a multicenter clinical trial. TOAST. Trial of Org 10172 in Acute Stroke Treatment. *Stroke* 1993; **24**: 35–41.

Barnett HJM, Mohr JP, Stein BM, Yatsu FM (Eds). *Stroke: Pathophysiology, Diagnosis & Management*. Churchill Livingstone, London, 1998.

Di Tullio MR, Homma S. Mechanisms of cardioembolic stroke. *Curr Cardiol Rep* 2002; **4**: 141–8.

Khrenov AV, Ananyeva NM, Griffin JH, Saenko EL. Coagulation pathways in atherothrombosis. *Trends Cardiovasc Med* 2002; **12**: 317–24.

Kitagawa Y, Okayasu H, Matsuoka Y et al. Anticardiolipin antibody in cerebral infarction. *Rinsho Shinkeigaku* 1991; **31**: 391–5.

Kolominsky-Rabas PL, Weber M, Gefeller O et al. Epidemiology of ischemic stroke subtypes according to TOAST criteria: incidence, recurrence, and long-term survival in ischemic stroke subtypes: a population-based study. *Stroke* 2001; **32**: 2735–40.

Libman RB, Kwiatkowski TG, Hansen MD et al. Differences between anterior and posterior circulation stroke in TOAST. *Cerebrovasc Dis* 2001; **11**: 311–16.

Mann KG, Butenas S, Brummel K. The dynamics of thrombin formation. *Arterioscler Thromb Vasc Biol* 2003; **23**: 17–25.

Mitsias P, Levine SR. Large cerebral vessel occlusive disease in systemic lupus erythematosus. *Neurology* 1994; **44**: 385–93.

Murat Sumer M, Erturk O. Ischemic stroke subtypes: risk factors, functional outcome and recurrence. *Neurol Sci* 2002; **22**: 449–54.

Nendaz M, Sarasin FP, Bogousslavsky J. How to prevent stroke recurrence in patients with patent foramen ovale: anticoagulants, antiaggregants, foramen closure, or nothing? *Eur Neurol* 1997; **37**: 199–204.

Schmal M, Marini C, Carolei A *et al*. Different vascular risk factor profiles among cortical infarcts, small deep infarcts, and primary intracerebral haemorrhage point to different types of underlying vasculopathy. A study from the L'Aquila Stroke Registry. *Cerebrovasc Dis* 1998; **8**: 14–19.

3. General preventive measures

Primary prevention
High-risk groups

Primary prevention

Acute treatment of stroke will evolve and improve in the future. Nonetheless, prevention of strokes and transient ischaemic attacks (TIAs) remains the most important medical aspect in this area. There are several well documented risk factors for stroke that demand attention. Regular screening for these risk factors and appropriate management will reduce the subsequent chance of stroke. The American Heart Association have issued a scientific statement concerning primary prevention of ischaemic stroke and it contains useful advice.

> Regular screening for stroke risk factors (eg hypertension, atrial fibrillation and diabetes) and appropriate treatment can reduce the likelihood of suffering a stroke

Suggested management of well-documented modifiable risk factors is set out in Table 3.1. This table provides a suggested approach to the primary prevention of stroke. Clearly the implementation of protocols will be dependent on the local availability of resources and staff.

High-risk groups

Certain high-risk groups can be identified, including those with:

- previous TIA
- cardiovascular disease
- hypertension
- atrial fibrillation
- diabetes.

Efforts to screen for risk factors and institute primary prevention strategies can be concentrated on these high-risk individuals.

Patients with TIA should essentially be investigated and treated in the same way as those presenting with stroke, as outlined in Chapter 10. Patients with cardiovascular disease of all types are at an increased risk of stroke and risk factors for stroke, many of which are common to cardiovascular disease, need to be identified and treated. Hypertension is a major risk factor for stroke and in those patients with hypertension, other risk factors need to be identified and addressed as well as ensuring that the hypertension is adequately controlled. Patients with co-existing diabetes are at increased risk and careful attention should be paid to glucose levels and other risk factors.

> Both stroke and TIA patients should be investigated and treated in the same way

Less well-documented modifiable risk factors and suggested strategies for dealing with them in primary prevention are set out in Table 3.2.

> All modifiable risk factors should be targeted in the treatment and prevention of stroke, including less well-documented factors, eg obesity and control of inflammatory processes

Table 3.1
Common modifiable stroke risk factors and their primary prevention strategies

Factor	Goal	Recommendations
Hypertension	SBP <140 mmHg	Measure BP in all adults regularly. Especially important in older adults
	DBP <85 mmHg	Promote lifestyle modification: weight control, physical activity, moderation of alcohol intake, moderate sodium intake. If BP >140/90 mmHg after three months of life habit modification or if initial BP >180/100 mmHg, add antihypertensive medication. In primary prevention choose appropriate drug depending on individual patient
Smoking	Cessation	Strongly encourage patient and family to stop smoking. Provide counselling and formal programs as available. Nicotine replacement and bupropion for selected patients
Diabetes	Improved glucose control; treatment of hypertension and dyslipidaemia	Diet, oral hypoglycaemics or insulin as appropriate
Asymptomatic carotid stenosis		Patients with asymptomatic stenosis should be fully evaluated for other treatable causes of stroke. Asymptomatic carotid stenosis not considered for surgery in UK
Atrial fibrillation		
Age <65 years, no risk factors		Aspirin or warfarin
Age <65 years, with risk factors		Warfarin (target INR 2.5; range 2.0–3.0)
Age 65–75 years, no risk factors		Aspirin or warfarin
Age 65–75 years, with risk factors		Warfarin (target INR 2.5; range 2.0–3.0)
Age >75 years, with or without risk factors		Warfarin (target INR 2.5; range 2.0–3.0)
Lipids*		
Initial evaluation (no CHD)		
CHD event risk <30% over 10 years	Improve lipid profile	Lifestyle measures and reassess at 5 years
CHD event risk ≥30% over 10 years and TC <5 mmol/L	Improve lipid profile	Lifestyle measures and reassess annually
CHD event risk >30% over 10 years and TC >5 mmol/L	Improve lipid profile	Lifestyle measures and reassess in 3–6 months; take fasting level – if >5.0 mmol/L lipid-lowering therapy (target TC <5.0 mmol/L)

*Lipid reduction guidelines may become more strict for primary prevention
SBP, systolic blood pressure; DBP, diastolic blood pressure; CHD, coronary heart disease; TC, total cholesterol; INR, International Normalized Ratio

Table 3.2
Additional modifiable stroke risk factors and their primary prevention strategies

Factor	Goal	Suggested strategy
Obesity	Reduce weight/BMI to acceptable limits, ie BMI 20–25	Diet or counselling. Pharmacological strategies could be considered in appropriate circumstances (orlistat, sibutramine)
Physical inactivity	Minimize inactivity. Promote exercise for 30 minutes most days	Promote healthy lifestyle with exercise. Modify programme in light of comorbid conditions
Alcohol abuse	End abuse	Counselling, use of voluntary agencies (eg Alcoholics Anonymous), specialist psychiatric support, pharmacological agents in selected cases (disulfiram, acamprosate)
Hyperhomocysteinaemia	Reduce homocysteine levels	Increase fruit and vegetable intake, vitamin supplements with B12, folate, pyridoxine and betaine
Inflammatory processes	Reduce inflammation	Current data do not provide sufficient evidence for strategy

Further reading

Aronow WS. Management of the older person with atrial fibrillation. *J Gerontol A Biol Sci Med Sci* 2002; **57**: M352–63.

Chalmers J, Chapman N. Challenges for the prevention of primary and secondary stroke: the importance of lowering blood pressure and total cardiovascular risk. *Blood Press* 2001; **10**: 344–51.

Francos GC, Schairer HL Jr. Hypertension. Contemporary challenges in geriatric care. *Geriatrics* 2003; **58**: 44–9; quiz 50.

Goldstein LB, Adams R, Becker K *et al*. Primary prevention of ischemic stroke: A statement for healthcare professionals from the stroke council of the American Heart Association. *Stroke* 2001; **32**: 280–99.

Gorelick PB, Alter M (Eds). The Prevention of Stroke. CRC Press, 2002.

Hawkins BT, Brown RC, Davis TP. Smoking and ischemic stroke: a role for nicotine? *Trends Pharmacol Sci* 2002; **23**: 78–82.

Hennessy MJ, Britton TC. Transient ischaemic attacks: evaluation and management. *Int J Clin Pract* 2000; **54**: 432–6.

Kernan WN, Inzucchi SE, Viscoli CM *et al*. Insulin resistance and risk for stroke. *Neurology* 2002; **9**: 809–15.

Messinger-Rapport BJ, Sprecher D. Prevention of cardiovascular diseases. Coronary artery disease, congestive heart failure, and stroke. *Clin Geriatr Med* 2002; **18**: 463–83.

Vinik A, Flemmer M. Diabetes and macrovascular disease. *J Diabetes Complications* 2002; **16**: 235–45.

4. Diagnosis and evaluation of stroke

Differential diagnosis
Signs and symptoms of stroke
Classification
Severity of stroke
Signs and symptoms of TIAs
Prognosis in TIA

Differential diagnosis

When a patient has an acute neurological insult it is crucial that an accurate diagnosis is made. The differential diagnosis of stroke and transient ischaemic attack (TIA) is wide and attention to aspects of the history and examination are very important. Important differential diagnoses are shown in Table 4.1.

Table 4.1
Differential diagnosis of acute stroke – including other causes of acute neurological deficit(s)

- Epileptic seizure and postictal
- Structural lesions
- Subdural haematoma
- Tumour (1°, 2°)
- Metabolic/toxic
  - Hyponatraemia
  - Hypocalcaemia
  - Hepatic encephalopathy
  - Wernick–Korsakoff syndrome
  - Hypoglycaemia
  - Hyperglycaemia
  - Alcohol and drugs
- Head injury
- Encephalitis/cerebral abscess
- Hypertensive encephalopathy
- Multiple sclerosis
- Creutzfeld–Jakob disease
- Peripheral nerve lesion
- Functional

Features of a cerebral infarction

The majority of strokes are due to cerebral infarction. It is often difficult, if not impossible, to distinguish from haemorrhage on clinical grounds alone. Features suggestive of cerebral infarction include:

- history of TIAs
- stuttering stroke
- moderate headache
- consciousness relatively unaffected
- atrial fibrillation
- other risk factors, eg atherosclerosis, age
- carotid bruits
- clinical evidence of internal carotid artery occlusion, eg retinal signs.

Thrombosis and embolism are the main mechanisms. The precise effects depend upon the arterial territory affected.

> Most strokes are caused by cerebral infarction due to embolism or thrombosis

Features of a cerebral haemorrhage

Haemorrhagic strokes are most often associated with hypertension and cerebral aneurysms. They can occur during activity with no history of any previous attack. Without diagnostic testing they can be impossible to differentiate from an infarction.

Features suggestive of haemorrhage:

- sudden onset – no prodrome
- occurrence during waking hours
- severe headache, vomiting, early onset of coma
- progression of deficit, eg loss of consciousness
- recognized risk factors, especially hypertension
- increased International Normalized Ratio.

It is only possible to distinguish between haemorrhagic strokes and cerebral infarctions by carrying out imaging. This must be done soon after the event

Other considerations

In addition to accurately diagnosing a stroke or TIA, the general condition of the individual patient must be taken into account. The following must be considered for every patient:

- Is there a life-threatening concomitant disease?
- What kind of stroke is this?
- Where in the brain is it?
- What is the aetiology (is it likely to be atherosclerosis related, cardio-embolic, haemodynamic or are there small-vessel lesions)?
- How dangerous is the stroke (are there signs of poor prognosis)?

An initial idea about stroke aetiology is derived from the neurovascular examination, which focuses on the neck vessels, the intracranial vessels and the heart. Stroke severity and prognosis in ischaemic stroke are, in general, correlated with the severity of the neurologic deficit and the presence or absence of very early ischaemic changes on the initial computerized tomography scan. Dense hemiplegia, forced eye deviation and decreased level of consciousness predict poor outcome. It is vital that imaging is carried out as soon as possible after the event.

Clinical examinations should be concerned with the nervous system, the heart and the neck vessels

Signs and symptoms

Symptoms at presentation of an acute stroke may be diverse and are not confined to weakness. Certain patterns of symptomatology are recognized, as shown in Table 4.2.

Table 4.2
Symptoms of stroke

- Loss of movement (paralysis) of any body area, including facial paralysis
- Weakness
- Decreased sensation
- Numbness
- Tingling or other sensation changes
- Decreased vision
- Language difficulties (dysphasia/aphasia)
  - slurred, thick, difficult speech
  - inability to speak
  - inability to understand speech
  - may have difficulty with reading or writing
- Inability to recognize or identify sensory stimuli (agnosia) resulting in 'neglect' of one side of the body
- Loss of memory
- Vertigo (abnormal sensation of movement)
- Loss of coordination
- Swallowing difficulties
- Personality changes
- Mood/emotion changes (such as depression or apathy)
- Consciousness changes
  - sleepiness
  - stuporous/somnolent/lethargic
  - comatose/unconscious
- Urinary incontinence (lack of control over bladder)
- Lack of control over the bowels
- Cognitive decline
  - dementia
  - easily distracted
  - impaired judgment
  - limited attention

Additional symptoms

There are other additional symptoms that are associated with acute stroke, but on their own are not necessarily diagnostic. These symptoms include unpredictable (jerky), uncontrollable or dysfunctional movement, which can embrace uncontrollable eye movements as well as limb movement. Signs in the face include tongue problems, drooling and eye-lid drooping. An abnormal lack of sweating is sometimes seen, as is a temporary absence of breathing. Patients can present with fatigue, fainting episodes or possibly even seizures and generally strange or unusual behaviour can also result from stroke.

Classification

Stroke syndromes can be categorized by the Oxford Community Stroke Project classification (OCSP) or by the Trial of Org 10172 in Acute Stroke Treatment (TOAST) criteria.

Oxfordshire Community Stroke Project classification

Common stroke syndromes can be classified according to the Oxfordshire Community Stroke Project (OCSP) classification. This uses an anatomical method based on arterial supply to clinically define the type of stroke. This is illustrated in Figure 4.1 where computerized tomography (CT) scan appearances augment the clinical classification, defining whether the stroke is due to a haemorrhage or an infarct:

- TACS – total anterior circulation stroke
- PACS – partial anterior circulation stroke
- LACS – lacunar stroke
- POCS – posterior circulation stroke

The 'S' for 'stroke' or 'syndrome' is often substituted with an 'I' if an infarct has occurred, ie TACI, PACI, LACI, POCI.

> The OCSP classification divides common stroke syndromes in to four classes: TACS, PACS, LACS and POCS. Scanning defines whether an infarct or haemorrhage has occurred

The OCSP clinical classification is a useful way of clinically defining stroke by assessing each stroke patient carefully. The features of a total anterior circulation stroke (TACS) are shown in Table 4.3. This syndrome is associated with a poorer outcome than the partial anterior stroke syndrome (PACS) – whose clinical features are set out in Table 4.4 – principally because a larger area of the brain has been damaged in TACS. Lacunar strokes have no higher functional abnormalities and by definition represent small (<1.5 cm) areas

of brain damage. Their features are set out in Table 4.5. They are usually infarcts but careful imaging by magnetic resonance imaging (MRI) scans can reveal small haemorrhages. Table 4.6 shows the clinical features of the posterior circulation stroke (POCS). These can affect the occipital cortex, the cerebellum or the brain stem, and have various effects. Examples of this type of stroke include the lateral medullary syndrome and there are many with different eponyms.

Table 4.3
TACS: total anterior circulation stroke

TACS usually has the following features simultaneously:
- Higher dysfunction depending on hemisphere involved this may be
    - dysphasia, often left hemisphere
    - visuospatial, often right hemisphere
- Homonymous hemianopia
- Motor/sensory deficit in ≥2/3 face/arm/leg on one side of the body

---

Table 4.4
PACS: partial anterior circulation stroke

ANY ONE of these features may be present:
- Two out of three clinical features of TACS
    - higher dysfunction
        → dysphasia
        → visuospatial
    - homonymous hemianopia
    - motor/sensory deficit in ≥2/3 face/arm/leg on one side of the body
- Higher dysfunction alone
- Limited motor/sensory deficit

Table 4.5
LACS: lacunar stroke

ANY ONE of these:
- Pure motor stroke (≥2/3 face/arm/leg)
- Pure sensory stroke (≥2/3 face/arm/leg)
- Sensorimotor stroke (≥2/3 face/arm/leg)
- Ataxic hemiparesis
A lacunar stroke would HAVE NONE of these:
- New dysphasia
- New visuospatial problem
- Proprioceptive sensory loss only
- No vertebrobasilar features

a)

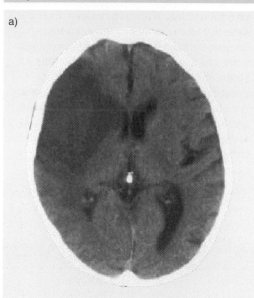

b)

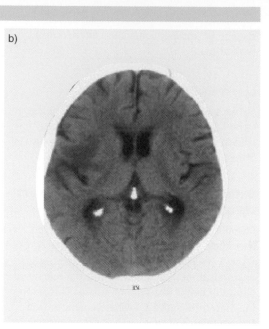

c)

d)

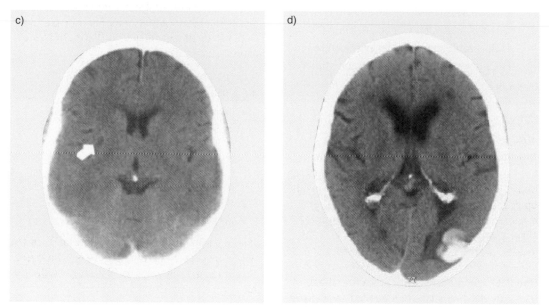

Figure 4.1
CT scans from patients in the database showing typical features of the Bamford or Oxfordshire Community Stroke Project classification of stroke subtypes. a) TACS, total anterior circulation syndrome (infarction); b) PACS, posterior anterior circulation syndrome (infarction); c) LACS, lacunar syndrome (infarction); d) POCS, posterior circulation syndrome (haemorrhage).

Table 4.6
POCS: posterior circulation stroke

ANY OF THESE FEATURES:
- Cranial nerve palsy on one side of the body
AND
- Contralateral motor/sensory deficit
OR
- Bilateral motor OR sensory deficit
- Conjugate eye movement problems
- Cerebellar dysfunction WITHOUT ipsilateral long tract signs
- Isolated homonymous hemianopia

The TOAST criteria

The TOAST classification denotes five subtypes of ischaemic stroke:

- large-artery atherosclerosis
- cardioembolism
- small-vessel occlusion
- stroke of other determined aetiology
- stroke of undetermined aetiology.

The categorization depends on the clinical features and results of investigations.

Other types of stroke

Stuttering stroke

A stuttering stroke may occur with occlusion of the internal carotid artery. The actual impact of occlusion of the internal carotid artery depends upon the effectiveness of compensatory mechanisms, principally the circle of Willis. (The circle of Willis is a vascular structure located on the floor of the cranial cavity and represents the termination of the basilar and internal carotid arteries. The circle of Willis loops around the brain stem above the pons and the brain's major blood vessels [the anterior, middle and posterior cerebral arteries] branch from it. Because the circle of Willis is supplied by three vessels, damage to one may not compromise the blood supply to the brain as the arrangement allows collateral flow. In addition, even if there is an occlusion of part of the circle itself, blood can flow in either direction around it.) It also depends on the

external carotid, which may provide flow to the anterior and the middle cerebral arteries through meningeal branches, and retrogradely through the ophthalmic artery to the internal carotid. Total occlusion may be silent or catastrophic. Characteristically, the picture is one of a stuttering stroke. If the innominate artery is occluded after branching from the aortic arch, a similar picture may be seen. Additionally, there will be reduced blood pressure in the right arm.

> Stuttering stroke occurs when the internal carotid artery is occluded, but the stroke impact depends on compensatory mechanisms, eg the circle of Willis, and alternative routes of blood flow

Severity of stroke

Various standardized tests can be used to assess the severity of stroke. For example, the National Institutes of Health (NIH) stroke scale assesses the domains of:

- consciousness
- vision
- extraocular movements
- facial palsy
- limb strength
- ataxia
- sensation
- speech
- language.

It uses 15 items scored from 0 to 2 or 3. In the NIH stroke scale higher scores reflect increased severity of the deficit; the highest possible total score is 42.

Signs and symptoms of TIAs

Diagnosis of transient ischaemic attacks can be problematic. They may be overdiagnosed by generalists and others who assume labelling unusual or undiagnosed non-specific or non-focal neurological symptoms as a TIA is satisfactory. The lifetime incidence of TIA is around 4%. Because the symptoms of TIAs last for less than 24 hours and typically less than one hour, it must be borne in mind that other neurological diseases can cause transient symptoms. These diseases include focal fits, migraine and space-occupying lesions.

> Symptoms of transient ischaemic attack last for less than 24 hours and normally under one hour, thereby making diagnosis difficult. Also, certain neurological diseases can cause transient TIA-like symptoms

Common symptoms

Common symptoms of TIAs are shown in Table 4.7.

Table 4.7
Symptoms of TIAs

Carotid distribution (80%)
- Unilateral motor/sensory defects
- Dysphasia
- Amaurosis fugax
- Homonymous hemianopia
- Combinations of the above

Vertebrobasilar (20%)
- Motor/sensory deficits affecting any combination of extremities (including crossed face and limbs, bilateral, may change from side to side in different attacks)
- Ataxia
- Homonymous hemianopia
- Bilateral visual loss
- The following in combination with one another or any of the above symptoms, but NOT in isolation:
  - vertigo
  - diplopia
  - dysphagia
  - dysarthria
- Combination of the above

Symptoms that do not justify the diagnosis of TIA

Certain neurological symptoms do not by themselves usually constitute a diagnosis of TIA. These are listed in Table 4.8.

There are numerous causes of transient focal neurological attacks. Reasons behind such

Table 4.8
Symptoms that do not justify the diagnosis of TIA

- Loss of consciousness
- Falls
- Confusion
- Generalized weakness
- Dizziness
- Incontinence
- Amnesia
- Sensory symptoms confined to part of one limb or face

attacks include stroke or TIA, migraine aura, partial seizures, transient global amnesia, multiple sclerosis, labyrinthine disorders, peripheral nerve lesions and myasthenia gravis. Transient focal neurological attacks can also occur as a result of intracranial structural lesions (eg tumour, giant aneurysm, arteriovenous malformation, chronic subdural haematoma), metabolic disturbances (eg hypoglycaemia, hyperglycaemia, hypercalcemia, hyponatraemia) and psychological problems (eg hyperventilation, panic, somatization disorder).

Prognosis in TIA

A study of 1707 patients presenting to an emergency department with a TIA has revealed how serious they are. At three months, 10.5% of the patients had sustained a stroke and 2.6% had died. A spectrum of stroke risk ranged from 0–34%. Independent risk factors identified were age >60 years, diabetes mellitus, a TIA lasting over 10 minutes, weakness and speech impairment. The long-term outlook after a TIA is not good. The risk of stroke is 11.6% at one year and 30% at five years. The risk of myocardial infarction is high, with an annual incidence of 2.4%. Coronary heart disease is the commonest cause of death and, with a mortality of 6.3% per year, it is higher than in unselected patients with stable angina and similar to that in patients with stable angina treated medically and those with three-vessel coronary disease.

Non-lacunar and non-retinal TIAs (or unselected TIA patients) are at twice the risk of vascular events than patients with lacunar TIAs or amaurosis fugax. Hemispheric TIAs and underlying carotid stenosis >70% carry a risk of stroke of 42% within two years.

> Long-term prognosis after TIA is poor; many people go on to suffer stroke, myocardial infarction or coronary heart disease, and 2.6% of TIA sufferers die within three months

Further reading

A classification and outline of cerebrovascular diseases. II. *Stroke* 1975; **6**: 564–616.

Adams HP Jr, Bendixen BH, Kappelle LJ *et al.* Classification of subtype of acute ischemic stroke. Definitions for use in a multicenter clinical trial. TOAST. Trial of Org 10172 in Acute Stroke Treatment. *Stroke* 1993; **24**: 35–41.

Bamford J. Clinical examination in diagnosis and subclassification of stroke. *Lancet* 1992; **339**: 400–2.

Bogousslavsky J, Caplan L (Eds). *Stroke Syndromes.* Cambridge University Press: Cambridge, 1995.

Bosworth HB. Trends in stroke mortality: the impact of the Year 2000 Age Standard and the International Statistical Classification of Diseases and Related Health Problems, 10th Revision. *Stroke* 2002; **33**: 1722.

Johnston SC, Gress DR, Browner WS, Sidney S. Short-term prognosis after emergency department diagnosis of TIA. *JAMA* 2000; **284**: 2901–6.

Libman RB, Kwiatkowski TG, Hansen MD *et al.* Differences between anterior and posterior circulation stroke in TOAST. *Cerebrovasc Dis* 2001; **11**: 311–16.

Murat Sumer M, Erturk O. Ischemic stroke subtypes: risk factors, functional outcome and recurrence. *Neurol Sci* 2002; **22**: 449–54.

Odderson IR. The National Institutes of Health Stroke Scale and its importance in acute stroke management. *Phys Med Rehabil Clin N Am* 1999; **10**: 787–800.

Samuelsson M, Soderfeldt B, Olsson GB. Functional outcome in patients with lacunar infarction. *Stroke* 1996; **27**: 842–6.

Sturmer T, Schlindwein G, Kleiser B *et al.* Clinical diagnosis of ischemic versus hemorrhagic stroke: applicability of existing scores in the emergency situation and proposal of a new score. *Neuroepidemiology* 2002; **21**: 8–17.

5. Imaging

Computerized tomography scanning
Magnetic resonance imaging
Magnetic resonance angiography
Doppler carotid scans
Intima-media thickness measurement
Other imaging techniques

To manage stroke patients effectively there needs to be diagnostic imaging machinery readily available.

Computerized tomography scanning

Usually, after blood tests have been ordered, the first test will be (cranial) computerized tomography (CT) scanning. Non-contrast CT scanning will establish the differential diagnosis between an intracerebral haemorrhage and acute ischaemic stroke. In addition, other intracranial pathologies will be defined using CT such as:

- an abscess
- a tumour, primary or secondary
- encephalitis
- sinus venous thrombosis
- occasionally unexpected subarachnoid haemorrhage.

> Computerized tomography scanning is the first imaging test done after a stroke. It can distinguish between acute ischaemic stroke and intracerebral haemorrhage if carried out within the first seven days after the event

Considerable expertise in the assessment of subtle early infarctions is essential to identify patients who may be treated with thrombolytic drugs, and also to identify patients with bad prognoses who are at risk of secondary haemorrhage and herniation.

Although CT scanning may not be very sensitive for early ischaemia (<6 hours), several findings can suggest ischaemic changes relatively early in the time course of stroke. These include loss of the grey–white matter interface, loss of sulci and loss of the insular ribbon.

Computerized tomography provides axial cross-sectional representations of the body according to the X-ray density of the tissues. At each level to be visualized, the X-ray source and detector record the penetration of a narrow beam of X-rays through a 180 degree arc around the patient. From this data a computer is able to reconstruct the cross-section of the body.

Cranial CT is good for supratentorial pathology but bone artefact limits the quality of views in the posterior fossa. The advantages of cranial CT scan include the quick speed and the ability to differentiate intracranial haemorrhage from infarction. Disadvantages in the assessment of ischaemic stroke include the fact that CT scans are best done promptly, preferably within 48 hours of, and no later than seven days after, the onset of symptoms. The full extent of infarcted tissue cannot be defined until several days afterwards, furthermore there may be a period where the infarct appears isodense at or around day three, so repeat scans are essential to determine prognosis. In certain cases, contrast media may be injected to improve visualization but this increases complexity and risk. The brainstem structures are poorly displayed because of bony artefacts. A disadvantage in the assessment of haemorrhage is the difficulty in distinguishing primary cerebral haemorrhage from confluent haemorrhagic infarction.

Computerized tomography is indicated in the investigation of stroke and certainly where there is doubt about the diagnosis. This occurs with a gradual onset or progressive neurological signs, no clear focal neurological signs or if no clear history is available. It is indicated when there is a need to exclude cerebral haemorrhage – the scan must be done within 7 days of onset because signs of haemorrhage may disappear over this time. It is indicated if thrombolytic, anticoagulant or antiplatelet treatment is contemplated or being used when a stroke occurs; if carotid endarterectomy and/or angioplasty is planned; when there is a suspected cerebellar stroke with obstructive hydrocephalus; and when there is acute onset of unsteadiness with deterioration.

> Computerized tomography scanning is useful in ruling out cerebral haemorrhage – if it is performed within a short time of the acute event, a cerebral haemorrhage will show up as a hyperdense area on CT scanning. However, if the CT is delayed for more than one week after the acute stroke it is possible for the haemorrhage to be resorbed by the body. An erroneous diagnosis of cerebral infarction might be made, as effectively a hyperdense area will be left behind on the CT scan

The latest CT scanners allow 3-D constuctions to be made and can allow angiography and other techniques to be used. Xenon CT scan is a relatively new technique that complements the non-contrast head CT scan and provides quantitative measurement of regional blood flow. Computerized tomography angiography, although not performed regularly, can demonstrate the vascular occlusion and areas of perfusion deficits. There will be more development of CT scanning in the future.

Magnetic resonanace imaging

It is necessary to understand the principles used in magnetic resonance imaging (MRI) scanning. The body can be considered to be a mass of small randomly arranged magnets. These magnets represent the nuclei of hydrogen atoms (protons) which have polarity and thus are able to alter their orientation if they are

subjected to a strong magnetic field. MRI utilizes these properties in a three-stage process:

- Precession: some of the protons within a patient placed in the scanner become aligned along the axis of the magnetic field. When these protons become magnetized they then rotate and wobble (precess) around the magnetized field axis.

- Resonance: by altering the radiofrequency, the orientation of rotation and wobbling can be altered. Different types of radiofrequency pulse can be used to produce different types of emitted signal with different structures.

- Emission: once the radiofrequency pulse is turned off, the protons begin to lose their phase cohesion and this results in the emission of very small radiofrequency signals. The magnitude, phase, amplitude and frequency of these signals are detected by a magnetic resonance imager and used to generate an image.

Magnetic resonance imaging has not yet become part of a routine assessment of the acute stroke patient. Modern sequences are capable of visualizing vessels (MR angiography), to estimate brain perfusion (perfusion-weighted imaging [PWI]) or to assess early cytotoxic oedema (diffusion-weighted imaging [DWI]). In the future, combinations of these techniques, eg PWI/DWI, may play an important role in early stroke management. It is theoretically possible that PWI/DWI mismatch can identify potentially salvageable tissues. However, because of the time required by current scanners to carry out MRI scans, X-ray CT scanning remains the initial diagnostic test of choice in most cases because it is faster. In the acute situation, it is important in practice to identify those patients who have had a haemorrhagic stroke.

Magnetic resonance imaging scans are probably the investigation of choice for lesions in the brain stem and posterior fossa. MRI scanning may be a helpful adjunct to CT scanning when diagnosis is in doubt. This may be useful in demyelination, cerebral vasculitis and further assessment of tumours.

Magnetic resonance imaging can be used to identify ischaemic changes in the brain within 45 minutes of stroke onset, which suggests that further development of this technique may be very useful. In addition, MRI has been used to visualize carotid arteries and can detect:

- fibrous intimal thickening
- lipid deposits
- calcification
- recent intramural haemorrhage
- atheromatous debris.

This cannot be regarded as a routine use of MRI technology at present but serves to illustrate its future potential.

> Although not a routine use for MRI, these scans can detect fibrous intimal thickening, lipid deposits, calcification, intramural haemorrhage and atheromatous debris

Magnetic resonance angiography

Magnetic resonance angiography (MRA) can be used to identify lesions within extracranial vessels (eg carotid dissection, carotid stenosis) and intracranial vessels. Stenosis of the internal carotid artery at the siphon can be identified. Gadolinium injection is used for contrast. With the advent of MRA, formal angiography of the cerebral vessels is less frequently used. An exception may be in the treatment and investigation of arterioventricular malformations (AVM). For AVM, and indeed for subarachnoid haemorrhage due to aneurysms in the cerebral circulation, it is necessary to use formal angiography in the treatment phase (ie the insertion of coils).

Doppler carotid scans

High-resolution B-mode imaging has been improved to the extent that real-time ultrasonographic evaluation of plaque morphology is possible. Colour Doppler flow imaging is a technique that combines grey-scale imaging with two-dimensional Doppler flow information in real time. A single representative Doppler shift is encoded by hue or colour intensity. Colours may be red or blue depending on direction of flow. Decreased colour saturation conventionally represents Doppler shifts. Through the contrast this technique imparts to the vascular lumen, the plaque surface and configuration can be evaluated.

Power Doppler imaging is a new technique being evaluated. Colour and brightness are related to the number of red blood cells producing the Doppler shift. Noise can be reduced and, being less angle dependent, curving or tortuous vessels may be seen more clearly. Compound imaging uses ultrasound beams specially steered at different angles and computer algorithms are used to produce clearer pictures.

Further development of Doppler carotid scans will include the characterization of plaque motion and four-dimensional colour Doppler flow imaging.

In many centres the quality of Doppler imaging is so good that the vascular surgeons do not require further investigation before carotid endarterectomy is carried out.

In certain instances, a *transcranial Doppler* can be performed, and this may be very valuable in identifying thrombosed middle cerebral or other arteries. This technique requires specialist equipment which can be portable and is sometimes used in Europe although rarely in the UK at present.

> Doppler imaging can be so clear that surgeons have no need to carry out further tests before they perform a carotid endarterectomy

Intima-media thickness measurement

Intima-media thickness (IMT) can be measured by B-mode ultrasound. This is a potential independent predictor of stroke risk. It is clearly related to age and appears to be an independent risk factor for atherogenesis. Further research will be carried out with this technique and it may become routine practice in the future.

> Intima-media thickness is related to age and is a risk factor for atherogenesis; it may be a predictor of stroke risk

Other imaging techniques

Many other imaging techniques continue to be developed. For example, the use of single proton emission computerized tomography (SPECT) in stroke is still relatively experimental and is only available at certain institutions. It is used to define areas of altered regional blood flow.

Further reading

Calliada F, Verga L, Pozza S et al. Selection of patients for carotid endarterectomy: the role of ultrasound. *J Comput Assist Tomogr* 1999; **23 (Suppl 1):** S75–81.

Fathi R, Marwick TH. Noninvasive tests of vascular function and structure: why and how to perform them. *Am Heart J* 2001; **141:** 694–703.

Goldmann A, Mohr W, Widder B. Tissue characterisation of atherosclerotic carotid plaques by MRI. *Neuroradiology* 1995; **37:** 631–5.

Gronholdt ML. B-mode ultrasound and spiral CT for the assessment of carotid atherosclerosis. *Neuroimaging Clin N Am* 2002; **12:** 421–35.

Hennerici M. *Imaging in Stroke*. Remedica Publishing: London, 2003.

Hennerici M, Meairs S. Imaging arterial wall disease. *Cerebrovasc Dis* 2000; **10 (Suppl 5):** 9–20.

Hoggard N, Wilkinson ID, Paley MN, Griffiths PD. Imaging of haemorrhagic stroke. *Clin Radiol* 2002; **57:** 957–68.

Luypaert R, Boujraf S, Sourbron S, Osteaux M. Diffusion and perfusion MRI: basic physics. *Eur J Radiol* 2001; **38:** 19–27.

Management soon after a stroke. *Drug Ther Bull* 1998; **36:** 51–4.

Moonis M, Fisher M. Imaging of acute stroke. *Cerebrovasc Dis* 2001; **11:** 143–50.

Sarkarati D, Reisdorff EJ. Emergent CT evaluation of stroke. *Emerg Med Clin N Am* 2002; **20:** 553–81.

Symons SP, Cullen SP, Buonanno F et al. Noncontrast conventional computed tomography in the evaluation of acute stroke. *Semin Roentgenol* 2002; **37:** 185–91.

Welch KM, Cao Y, Nagesh V. Magnetic resonance assessment of acute and chronic stroke. *Prog Cardiovasc Dis* 2000; **43:** 113–34.

6. Further hospital management

Clinical assessment
Stroke evaluation
Investigations

Clinical assessment

Clinical assessment of a patient with stroke or transient ischaemic attack (TIA) must be comprehensive. A full history should be taken, noting accurate timing of the onset of symptoms, the rate of development, risk factors for stroke and pre-morbid function. Important points to consider when taking a patient's history are shown in Table 6.1.

Table 6.1
Important points to note when taking the patient's history

- Onset
- Record time and rate of onset
- Risk factors, eg previous stroke, TIA, hypertension, ischaemic heart disease, peripheral arterial disease, diabetes, hyperlipidaemia, smoking, alcohol intake
- Check pre-stroke function – this can be affected by previous stroke or other important comorbidity, eg heart disease, respiratory disease, arthritis. It is unlikely that a patient will recover and rehabilitate to a better state than they were at prior to their current stroke
- Use recommended scales (see Appendix II)
  - Activities of Daily Living (ADL) – walking, stairs, transferring, bathing, dressing, grooming, toileting, feeding
  - Instrumental (or Extended) Activities of Daily Living (IADL) – shopping, cooking, driving, etc
- Employment
- Hobbies
- Use of help services at home

Stroke evaluation

The general assessment of a patient with a stroke or TIA should include the nutritional status, pulse (rate and rhythm), blood pressure, cardiac examination, examining the peripheral circulation and checking for carotid bruits. Table 6.2 is a suggested schema.

Table 6.2
General assessment of a stroke patient

- Nutritional status
- Pulse
- Blood pressure
- Cardiac examination (murmurs, heart failure)
- Peripheral circulation
- Carotid bruits
- Respiratory function

The neurological examination of a stroke or TIA patient should be thorough and will include measures of level of consciousness (possibly using the Glasgow coma scale – unconscious patients are at risk of aspiration and have a poorer outcome); eye movements (Doll's eye manoeuvre abnormal – suggest poor outcome, incoordination of eyes may suggest brain stem lesion); trunk control (ability to sit unaided is a useful prognostic sign) and incoordination (this can be impaired in cerebellar strokes and in certain lacunar strokes – this can not be assessed whan there is a weakness in the repective limb). Analysis of gait is also important. Swallowing assessment is required before any patient is allowed to swallow foods or fluids because the risk of aspiration is high. Visual field defects can occur and must be noted. Patients may have sensory loss in the affected side and there may also be sensory inattention, which can hinder recovery (as can visuospatial problems). These are set out in Table 6.3.

Investigations

Some important investigations are shown in Table 6.4. Investigations are aimed at clearly identifying the pathophysiological process of

Table 6.3

Neurological assessment of a stroke patient

- Level of consciousness
- Eye movements
- Limb power
- Communication
- Trunk control
- Gait
- Swallowing
- Mental test score
- Visuospatial function
- Visual fields
- Sensory testing

Table 6.4

Important investigations to be carried out after stroke or TIA

- CT scan or MRI scan
- Haemoglobin
- White blood cell count
- Platelets
- Lipids
- Glucose
- Urea, creatinine, electrolytes
- ECG
- Echocardiogram
- Carotid Doppler scan
- Blood pressure, ABPM
- Syphilis serology
- Auto-antibodies
- Clotting factors
- Genetic factors

CT, computerized tomography; MRI, magnetic resonance imaging; ECG, electrocardiogram; ABPM, ambulatory blood pressure monitoring

stroke (infarct or haemorrhage) and include imaging (computerized tomography [CT] or magnetic resonance imaging [MRI]) and detecting risk factors. Blood tests should include full blood count, tests for inflammation (plasma viscosity, erythrocyte sedimentation rate, C-reactive protein), renal function and electrolytes, glucose and lipids. An electrocardiogram might show atrial fibrillation, recent myocardial infarction, left ventricular hypertrophy or other cardiac abnormality. Echocardiography may be helpful in detecting potential sources of emboli or patent foramen ovale, although a transesophageal echocardiogram may be needed for these. Carotid duplex Doppler should be done on patients with carotid distribution cerebral infarcts to detect atheromatous lesions, as they may be operable. Transcranial Doppler can be used to demonstrate cerebral arterial blockage. Blood pressure assessment, including 24-hour ambulatory monitoring can be helpful, particularly in out-patients. Syphilis serology, auto-antibody tests (including rheumatoid, antinuclear and antiphospholipid antibodies), clotting factor (to detect possible thrombophilia) and genetic factor testing are often reserved for special circumstances, such as in younger patients with strokes who do not have 'traditional' risk factors, or in those with evidence of inflammation.

Investigations may be directed at identifying specific pathophysiological subtypes of stroke

and stroke risk factors for management and prognosis. Investigations that might contribute to these goals include:

- full blood count – for anaemia, polycythaemia, thrombocytopaenia
- sickle cell screen (if indicated)
- erythrocyte sedimentation rate, auto-antibodies (for vasculitis, collagen vascular disease); anticardiolipin antibodies, antinuclear antibody and rheumatoid factor may be required
- blood glucose (for hyperglycaemia in diabetes mellitus); if the random glucose is elevated then fasting and two-hour post prandial glucose should be tested. Glycosylated haemoglobin (HbA1C) concentration may be required
- serum cholesterol (total, high-density lipoprotein, low-density lipoprotein) and triglycerides – hyperlipidaemia
- plasma electrophoresis, viscosity studies in myeloma
- in younger patients a thrombophilia may be suspected and protein C, protein S, antithrombin III, factor VIII and fibrinogen

may be measured. Genetic testing for factor V Leiden (resistance to activated protein C) and for prothrombin 20210A>G mutation. Arterial thrombosis is not thought to be associated with these clotting abnormalities but further work is required. Venous thrombosis may be increased and an embolism can occur through a patent foramen ovale (transcranial doppler or transesophageal echocardiography may be required to establish this diagnosis). Fasting homocysteine may also be tested in this group

- Other genetic tests as indicated, eg CADASIL (Cerebral Autosomal Dominant Arteriopathy with Subcortical Infarcts and Leukoencephalopathy).
- other blood tests as indicated, eg neurosyphilis
- blood culture (if suspected infective endocarditis)
- chest X-ray (cardiac enlargement in hypertension or valvular disease)
- electrocardiogram (ventricular enlargement and/or arrhythmias in hypertensive/embolic disease; recent MI in embolic disease; conduction defect – embolic/output failure)
- retinal examination (retinopathy in hypertension, diabetes, embolic disease)
- urine analysis (polyarteritis, thrombocytopaenia)

- cervical spine X ray (will indicate atlanto-axial subluxation).

Further reading

Adams R, Acker J, Alberts M *et al.* Recommendations for improving the quality of care through stroke centers and systems: an examination of stroke center identification options: multidisciplinary consensus recommendations from the Advisory Working Group on Stroke Center Identification Options of the American Stroke Association. *Stroke* 2002; **33**: e1–7.

Bamford J. Assessment and investigation of stroke and transient ischaemic attack. *J Neurol Neurosurg Psychiatry* 2001; **70 (Suppl 1)**: I3–I6.

Cohen SN. *Management of Ischemic Stroke*. McGraw Hill: New York, 2000.

Harwood RH, Ebrahim S. A comparison of the responsiveness of the Nottingham extended activities of daily living scale, London handicap scale and SF-36. *Disabil Rehabil* 2000; **22**: 786–93.

Lawton MP. Instrumental Activities of Daily Living (IADL) Scale. Self-rated version. Incorporated in the Philadelphia Geriatric Center. Multilevel Assessment Instrument (MAI). *Psychopharmacol Bull* 1988; **24**: 789–91.

Mahoney FJ, Barthel DW. Functional evaluation: Barthel Index. *MD State Med J* 1965; **14**: 61–5.

Ronning OM, Guldvog B. Should stroke victims routinely receive supplemental oxygen? A quasi-randomized controlled trial. *Stroke* 1999; **30**: 2033–7.

Taylor CL, Selman WR. Emergency management of ischemic stroke. *Neurosurg Clin N Am* 2000; **11**: 365–75.

Wade DT, Collin C. The Barthel ADL index: a standard measure of physical disability? *Int Disabil Stud* 1988; **10**: 64–7.

7. Treatment of acute stroke

General principles
Treatment of haemorrhagic stroke
Treatment of ischaemic stroke

General principles

The acute management of stroke begins with the patient and their carers being educated to identify the early signs and symptoms of stroke and raising public awareness of stroke as a medical emergency. A high priority needs to be given by the emergency services to those suspected of experiencing evolving stroke; rapid admission to hospital will be required if interventions such as thrombolysis are to be considered.

> Stroke is an emergency and should be treated as such. Any delay in treatment will result in further brain damage

Once the patient arrives at hospital, assessment both clinically and with the use of appropriate imaging techniques needs to be rapid and treatment commenced rapidly if the narrow time window for intervention with thrombolysis is to be utilized. Clearly not all patients will be suitable for interventions such as thrombolysis, however, those patients who might benefit are not always readily identifiable in the community setting. Moreover, prompt identification of those with ischaemic stroke will allow early intervention with antiplatelet agents. Neurosurgical intervention in selected cases will be facilitated by prompt and accurate investigation.

Assessment and general physiological management

Patients admitted with signs and symptoms of stroke need assessment of baseline neurological and physiological function. Assessment begins with examination of basic function using the principles of airway, breathing and circulation; the Glasgow coma scale should be documented as well as physiological parameters such as pulse rate, blood pressure, temperature and pulse-oximetry. An examination to identify focal neurological deficits should be performed along with a general clinical examination. The time of onset of symptoms should be documented and the family or carers may be particularly useful as many patients will have problems with expressive and receptive dysphasia. Similarly the remainder of the clinical history will need to be completed. Regular reappraisal of condition is essential.

> On admission to hospital, stroke patients need to have their baseline physiological and neurological functions assessed using clinical and imaging techniques. This is essential when determining if deterioration or improvement are occurring

In certain patients cardiac monitoring, pulse-oximetry, invasive monitoring of fluid balance (measurement of central venous pressure) etc. will be essential to ensure a good outcome. Automated monitoring of physiological variables in the acute phase is possible and may improve outcome.

General management of stroke patients comprises respiratory and cardiac care, fluid and metabolic management, blood pressure control and dealing with other related problems, eg treating raised intracranial pressure. In addition, general treatment of acute stroke patients also includes treating:

- seizures
- deep venous thrombosis
- pulmonary embolism
- aspiration pneumonia
- urinary and other infections
- decubitus ulcers.

Pulmonary function and airway protection

To preserve oxygenation and metabolic turnover in the marginal zone of the insult, the so-called penumbra, adequate blood oxygenation with normal respiratory function is required. Airway problems in stroke patients are sometimes seen in those patients with severe pneumonia, heart failure, extensive vertebrobasilar or hemispheric infarction, with large intracranial haemorrhages or in patients with sustained seizure activity following hemispheric stroke. Patients with chronic obstructive pulmonary disease sometimes experience an exacerbation.

> After stroke it is important to keep the penumbra well oxygenated and ventilation may be indicated

In patients with respiratory problems or severe strokes continuous monitoring with pulse oximetry is required and ventilation may be indicated, particularly if supplemental oxygenation fails to keep O_2 levels above 95%. The prognosis of stroke patients undergoing intubation is not as bad as reported previously with a one-year survival rate of about one-third of the patients.

Particular care to avoid aspiration is required in those with swallowing disturbances and impaired brain stem reflexes. Whether early placement of a nasogastric tube is beneficial or not is uncertain, but nutrition is important and may be vital to recovery.

Cardiac care and blood pressure management

Cardiac care is aimed at maintaining a normal rhythm and blood pressure to ensure a reasonable cerebral blood flow. Cardiac arrhythmias secondary to stroke are not unusual. Significant alterations in the ST segments and the T waves on the electrocardiogram (ECG) may appear in the acute phase, mimicking myocardial ischaemia. Cardiac enzymes can also be elevated after

stroke but troponin concentrations are unlikely to be high unless there is direct myocardial damage. Every stroke patient should have an initial ECG – if this is normal, continuous ECG monitoring is not usually required. However, those patients with haemodynamic instability or major stroke syndromes should be continuously monitored. When there are cardiac arrhythmias, it may be necessary to restore normal rhythm by using drugs, DC cardioversion or pacemaker insertion.

Sometimes a myocardial infarction (MI) will accompany a stroke. Sometimes there are few symptoms or signs to suggest this diagnosis co-exists with cerebral ischaemia.

Maintenance of normal blood pressure is important. To avoid hypotension and thus potential diminution of cerebral blood flow, the intravascular blood volume must be kept stable. Intravenous rehydration with normal saline is usually sufficient. Inotropic agents are rarely required. Dobutamine increases cardiac output without substantially affecting either heart rate or blood pressure. Dopamine may be particularly useful in patients with hypotension or renal insufficiency. Increases in cardiac output may increase cerebral perfusion in areas that have lost their autoregulative capacity after acute ischaemia. The central venous pressure should be maintained at approximately 8–10 cm H_2O, and its monitoring, although not frequently used in a normal ward, will give early warning of a volume deficiency or volume overload, which both have negative effects on cerebral perfusion.

Hypertension management

Blood pressure monitoring and treatment is a critical issue. There have been no satisfactory trials of antihypertensive therapy in the acute phase, although in secondary prevention, blood pressure reduction is recommended once the patient is stable. Blood pressure should not be aggressively reduced in every acute stroke patient. The treatment of hypertension is currently less aggressive – many patients with acute infarcts have elevated blood pressure and this raised blood pressure may reduce or resolve with time. There may be worries that treatment in this situation may result in overshoot, ie a dramatic fall in blood pressure. Furthermore, cerebral blood flow autoregulation may be defective in an area of an evolving infarction so that flow in the critical penumbra zone is passively dependent on the mean arterial pressure.

Certain recommendations in the acute phase do exist. In the National Institute of Neurological Disorders and Stroke (NINDS) thrombolytic trial, intravenous treatment with antihypertensive agents was used when the systolic pressure was ⩾180 mmHg and/or the diastolic pressure was ⩾110 mmHg.

There are few indications for immediate antihypertensive therapy in the first hour after symptom onset, eg to allow administration of thrombolytic drugs. Treatment may be appropriate in the setting of acute myocardial ischaemia (although extreme lowering of blood pressure is not good for patients with this condition), cardiac insufficiency, acute renal failure or acute hypertensive encephalopathy. If the computerized tomography scan has shown a haemorrhagic cause of stroke, such as subarachnoid haemorrhage, intracranial haemorrhage, or epidural or subdural haematoma, antihypertensive treatment may also be started.

> If a CT scan shows a haemorrhagic cause of stroke and the patient is hypertensive, antihypertensive medication may be indicated

Antihypertensive medications used in the acute phase should be carefully chosen. It is not clear which is the safest or best drug available. Compounds containing nitrates are used – sodium nitroprusside (in North America) and nitroglycerine (in Europe) are frequently recommended in the acute phase, although both are said to increase intracranial pressure. Other agents are also used, eg angiotensin-converting enzyme inhibitors, beta-blockers (labetalol) and clonidine. When using antihypertensive medication it is important to avoid abrupt falls in blood pressure as this can adversely affect the circulation to the brain.

Fluid and electrolyte management

Stroke patients should be managed so they have a balanced fluid and electrolyte status. This avoids reduction in plasma volume, raised haematocrit and impairment of rheologic properties of the blood ('sludging'). If there is evidence of raised intracerebral pressure, a slightly negative fluid balance (about 300–500 ml negative balance daily) is usually recommended.

The electrolytes should be monitored daily in the acute phase and substituted accordingly. Glucose infusions are not recommended. Uncontrolled volume replacement may lead to pulmonary oedema, cardiac decompensation and increased cerebral oedema. Periperal intravenous access is needed for initial fluid management and blood draws. On rare occasions central venous access is used; this allows higher concentrations to be administered provided that continuous ECG monitoring is available. Serious electrolyte abnormalities are rare in stroke. However, hyponatraemia may occur due to inadequate antidiuretic hormone secretion (SIADH syndrome) or due to excess release of atrial natriuretic factor. Inadequate antidiuretic hormone secreting syndrome is managed by fluid restriction or hypertonic saline. If this fails then demeclocycline may be tried. When excess atrial natriuretic factor is the cause, normovolaemia should be maintained. Rarely hyponatraemia occurs in patients with oral or nasogastric fluid maintenance. Inadequate antidiuretic hormone secreting syndrome and excess atrial natriuretic factor should be excluded. Oral supplemental sodium (slow sodium) or fludrocortisone may be required in these situations.

Although harmful electrolyte abnormalities are rare after stroke, hyponatraemia can occur due to excess release of atrial natriuretic factor or inadequate antidiuretic hormone secreting syndrome

Haemodilution

Reductions in blood viscosity and improvements in cerebral blood flow by isovolaemic haemodilution that lowers the haematocrit by 15% can occur. However, several large clinical trials of isovolaemic haemodilution have been unable to demonstrate a decline in mortality or disability with treatment. Hypervolaemic haemodilution has been examined in small randomized trials with conflicting results. The clinical benefit of haemodilution therapy has not been established and the possibility of excess brain oedema has not been excluded.

Glucose metabolism

There is increasing evidence that high blood glucose is detrimental to acute stroke patients. Indeed, many stroke patients are diabetics and sometimes diabetes mellitus is discovered for the first time after an ischaemic infarct has developed. A pre-existing diabetic metabolic derangement may be dramatically worsened in the acute phase of stroke and temporary insulin treatment may become necessary. High glucose levels are not advantageous in stroke – a blood glucose level of ≥ 10 mmol/L suggests that an insulin regime to correct this may be needed. If insulin is administered intravenously, consideration should be given to an increased potassium requirement.

Pre-existing diabetes can be severely worsened in the acute phase of stroke

In general, glucose infusions should be avoided in the intravenous rehydration of stroke patients, unless hypoglycaemia exists. Hypoglycaemia can rarely mimic an acute ischaemic infarction, and its focal signs are not always those of a seizure. When hypoglycaemia is detected, an infusion of 10–20% glucose may be required.

Body temperature

Fever negatively influences neurological outcome after stroke. Experimentally, fever increases infarct size. Infection is a risk factor for stroke, and many patients develop a stroke after infection. Investigation and appropriate treatment with antibiotics for infection is warranted. Antipyretics, such as paracetamol, are advocated to help deal with fever. In Europe trials are examining whether lowering body temperature by physical means (eg cooled intravenous infusions and cooling pads) is worthwhile.

Treatment of haemorrhagic stroke

The Surgical Treatment of Intracranial Haemorrhage (STICH) trial is ongoing and may provide information on the role of neurosurgical intervention in acute haemorrhagic stroke. In general, severe strokes are associated with large volume haematomas, patients are barely conscious and do poorly; patients with mild strokes that are associated with small volume haemorrhages do better. The intervention policy will depend on the proximity and availability of neurosurgical expertise. In all cases good clinical management of physiological variables is important and treatment of any underlying cause is undertaken. Antithrombotic medications are avoided. Recently, blood pressure reduction with an angiotensin-converting enzyme (ACE) inhibitor and diuretic combination (perindopril and indapamide) has been shown to be useful in preventing further events in cerebral haemorrhage survivors.

Survivors of cerebral haemorrhage should be given an ACE inhibitor and diuretic combination to lower blood pressure and decrease the chance of a further event

Treatment of ischaemic stroke

Thrombolysis

Thrombolytic therapy with recombinant tissue plasminogen (rtPA) has given hope that emergency treatment can improve outcome in carefully selected patients. Thrombolytic therapy with rtPA (0.9 mg/kg body weight) given within three hours of stroke onset to patients with acute ischaemic stroke significantly improves outcome after stroke. This treatment is approved in North America and was approved in Europe in January 2003. There is some evidence that thrombolysis may also work up to six hours after stroke onset in carefully identified patients.

> Recombinant tissue plasminogen (rtPA) should be given in the ratio 0.9 mg/kg body weight within three hours of the onset of ischaemic stroke

The risks and benefits of this therapy are not undisputed. In certain parts of Europe, there is still some doubt about its risk:benefit ratio, which prevents some centres from actively promoting it. Problems obtaining CT scans at an early enough stage to permit the consideration of thrombolysis also exist. Caution is advised before giving intravenous rtPA to persons with severe stroke (NIH stroke scale >22), or if the CT demonstrates extended early changes of a major infarction, such as sulcal effacement, mass effect and oedema (this is in addition to the contra-indication of any evidence of haemorrhage). In centres where thrombolytic therapy is offered, it should only be given if the diagnosis is established by an experienced physician who has expertise in the diagnosis of stroke, and a CT of the brain is assessed by physicians who have expertise in reading this imaging study. Because the use of thrombolytic drugs carries the real risk of major bleeding, the risks and potential benefits of rtPA should be discussed whenever possible with the patient and family before treatment is initiated.

A recent meta-analysis of all randomized rtPA trials demonstrated an increase in independent patients without increased morbidity or mortality. According to the Cochrane reviewers, thrombolysis in acute ischaemic stroke seems to be increasingly robust within three and possibly six hours of stroke. However, the Cochrane reviewers still consider the number of patients randomized to be too small, so that there is little evidence on which subgroups of stroke patients might receive particular benefit or harm. Hence, there is not enough evidence to draw final conclusions about the effect of thrombolytic drugs in acute stroke. Currently intravenous administration of rtPA more than three hours after stroke should only be given as part of a clinical trial (eg International Stroke Trial 3 [IST3]).

Experience with other thrombolytic drugs is even more limited. Intravenous streptokinase has been shown to be associated with an unacceptable risk of haemorrhage and haemorrhage-associated death. Intra-arterial thrombolytic therapy of occlusions of the proximal part of the middle cerebral artery, using pro-urokinase, has been shown to be significantly associated with better outcome in a recently published randomized trial. This treatment requires superselective angiography and is only available in selected centres. The treatment is safe and efficacious in a six-hour time window.

Intra-arterial treatment of acute basilar occlusion with urokinase or rtPA is frequently used in selected centres, but has not been subjected to a randomized trial.

Other strategies using thrombolytic drugs or antiplatelet agents (glycoprotein IIa/IIb inhibitors) either on their own or in combination may eventually prove to be more effective than currently available treatments.

Defibrinogenating enzymes

Ancrod is a defibrinogenating enzyme derived from the Malayan pit viper. Recently, a European trial testing ancrod treatment in a six-hour time window has been terminated prematurely and further developmental work was abandoned because of adverse effects in the active treatment arm. One trial in America had previously shown that ancrod improved outcome after acute ischaemic stroke if given within three hours of stroke onset and over five days.

Antiplatelet drugs

Aspirin is indicated soon after an ischaemic stroke. It has been shown, in two very large randomized, non-blinded intervention studies (International Stroke Trial [IST], Chinese Acute Stroke Trial [CAST]) that aspirin given within 48 hours of stroke seems to reduce mortality and rate of recurrent stroke minimally, but statistically significantly. Whether the mild positive effect of early aspirin is due to an effect on the infarct itself or due to prevention of recurrent infarction is not yet clear. Aspirin has anti-inflammatory actions as well as antiplatelet effects and it is not known to what extent these properties are involved. Aspirin can probably be given soon after an acute stroke when CT scan or MRI scan is unavailable, since in the IST few patients later shown to have cerebral haemorrhage came to significant harm. Whether antiplatelet drugs other than aspirin (eg dipyridamole, clopidogrel) are indicated in the acute phase after acute ischaemic stroke is not known since there have been no studies in the acute phase.

> When given within 48 hours of ischaemic stroke, aspirin reduces mortality and risk of stroke recurrence

Heparin, heparinoids and low molecular weight heparin

Heparin as early anticoagulation has been used frequently in treatment after acute ischaemic stroke, particularly in Europe and the USA. Unfortunately, none of the trials that have been performed has supported the idea that early heparin may influence outcome after ischaemic stroke or at least may reduce the number of recurrent strokes. Heparinoids and low molecular weight heparins are more specific anticoagulants and obviate the need for careful continuous coagulation studies. Several studies that have used intravenous heparinoids, subcutaneous low molecular weight heparin or subcutaneous heparin failed to show an overall benefit of treatment. Although there was some kind of improvement in outcome or reduction in stroke recurrence rates, this was almost always counterbalanced by an increased number of haemorrhagic complications. In no case was superiority over aspirin therapy ever shown.

There have been no randomized studies in the past 10 years to compare the effects of early full anticoagulation with conventional heparin following acute ischaemic stroke. This is a pity as it is not known whether this is beneficial or detrimental.

It is believed that certain high-risk patients (such as patients with stroke associated with atrial fibrillation) should be studied separately. There is evidence that treatment with aspirin until warfarin becomes effective is as good as treatment with heparin. However, in the absence of data, the remaining indications for the use of acute heparin after ischaemic stroke are not evidence-based. Table 7.1 gives some indications as to when full-dose intravenous heparin or an alternative heparinoid or low molecular weight heparin may currently still be proposed.

Table 7.1
Indications for heparin, heparinoids or low molecular weight heparin treatment after stroke

- Stroke due to cardiac emboli with high risk of re-embolization (artificial valves, atrial fibrillation, myocardial infarction with mural thrombi, left atrial thrombosis)
- Coagulopathies such as protein C and S deficiency
- APC resistance
- Symptomatic dissection of extracranial arteries
- Symptomatic extra- and intracranial stenoses
  - symptomatic internal carotid stenosis prior to operation
  - crescendo TIAs or stroke in progression
- Sinus venous thrombosis

APC, activated protein C; TIA, transient ischaemic attack

When heparin itself is used it is usually recommended to elevate the partial thromboplastin time up to twice the individual baseline. Heparin should only be given as long as it takes to decide on the appropriate secondary prevention. Contra-indications for treatment with heparin include:

- large cerebral infarcts (more than 50% of middle cerebral artery territory)
- uncontrollable arterial hypertension
- advanced microvascular changes in the brain.

> Heparin should not be given when a patient has uncontrollable arterial hypertension, large cerebral infarcts or advanced microvascular changes in the brain

Neuroprotection

Despite many drugs from many classes having the potential to protect against ischaemic neuronal damage that occurs after an acute stroke, and many positive results in experimental animal models of ischaemic stroke, in clinical trials not one single neuroprotective agent has been shown to influence outcome after stroke. Serious side-effects and lack of efficacy have led to disappointment. Currently, there is no recommendation to treat patients with neuroprotective drugs after ischaemic stroke.

> Neroprotective drugs have not been shown to affect outcome after stroke

Further reading

CAST: randomised placebo-controlled trial of early aspirin use in 20,000 patients with acute ischaemic stroke. CAST (Chinese Acute Stroke Trial) Collaborative Group. *Lancet* 1997; **349**: 1641–9.

Pulsinelli WA, Levy DE, Sigsbee B *et al*. Increased damage after ischemic stroke in patients with hyperglycemia with or without established diabetes mellitus. *Am J Med* 1983; **74**: 540–4.

Saxena R, Lewis S, Berge E *et al*. Risk of early death and recurrent stroke and effect of heparin in 3169 patients with acute ischemic stroke and atrial fibrillation in the International Stroke Trial. *Stroke* 2001; **32**: 2333–7.

The International Stroke Trial (IST): a randomised trial of aspirin, subcutaneous heparin, both, or neither among 19,435 patients with acute ischaemic stroke. International Stroke Trial Collaborative Group. *Lancet* 1997; **349**: 1569–81.

Tissue plasminogen activator for acute ischemic stroke. The National Institute of Neurological Disorders and Stroke rt-PA Stroke Study Group. *N Engl J Med* 1995; **333**: 1581–7.

8. Secondary prevention of ischaemic stroke

Agents
Procedures

In any patient who has experienced a stroke or transient ischaemic attack (TIA) the prevention of a second, potentially devastating stroke is clearly a major priority. Another priority is the prevention of myocardial infarction, ischaemic heart disease or peripheral vascular disease which stroke patients are prone to developing. The range of risk factors predisposing to stroke is discussed in previous chapters. As more treatment modalities become available, a rational approach to assessing risk factors needs to be developed by each stroke centre and protocols must be developed to ensure patients receive optimal secondary preventive therapy. A considerable amount of information can be identified by obtaining a suitable history and performing a complete clinical examination, paying particular attention to cardiovascular and neurological signs and symptoms, although investigations will usually be required to complete the assessment (see

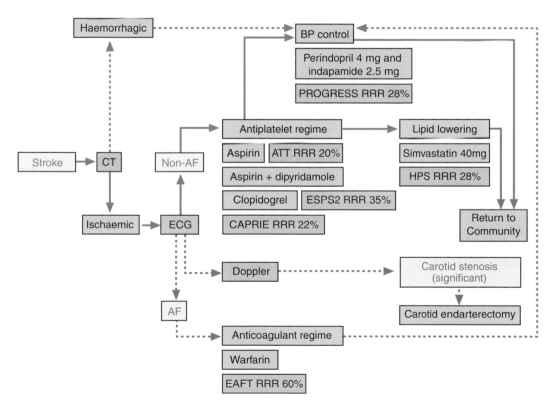

Figure 8.1
An example of a potential pathway for stroke secondary prevention.

BP, blood pressure; CT, computerized tomography; ECG, electrocardiogram; HPS, Heart Protection Study; RRR, relative risk reduction; CAPRIE, clopidogrel versus aspirin in patients at risk of ischaemic events; ATT, Antithrombotic Trialists; ESPS2, European Stroke Prevention Study 2; AF, atrial fibrillation

Chapter 6). Figure 8.1 shows one potential pathway for the investigation of a patient presenting with a stroke or TIA.

A large body of evidence is evolving which attests the value and efficacy of secondary prevention strategies. It is vital that all clinicians caring for stroke patients are aware of the current evidence so that they can make informed choices with their patients, taking in to account the risks and benefits of each preventive treatment. They should also be able to justify the resource implications for each treatment implemented.

> It is important the clinicians are aware of the latest evidence on preventive treatments for stroke so they can help their patients to make informed choices

Agents

Antiplatelet agents

Platelets physiologically aggregate at the site of endothelial damage to form a physical 'plug' to seal haemorrhaging vessels. Exposed collagen in vascular endothelium causes platelet aggregation. Rupture of the cap of atheromatous plaques also cause platelet adhesion and activation of inflammatory cascades leading to occlusion of the vessel; in the cerebral arterial system – this may result in stroke. This model for thrombotic stroke clearly identifies the role of platelets and this offers a therapeutic option to reduce the propensity for further stroke. One meta-analysis of the Antiplatelet Trialist's Collaboration found that antiplatelet therapy reduces the odds of non-fatal stroke by 23% in patients with a history of stroke or TIA.

> Antiplatelet therapy reduces the risk of non-fatal stroke by 23% in patients with a history of TIA or stroke

Aspirin was the first anti-platelet agent available and more recently other agents have been developed. Dipyridamole, Clopidogrel (and Ticlopidine) have different mechanisms of action from aspirin although each have a proven antiplatelet function. Aspirin remains the most commonly used antiplatelet agent; it is a cyclo-oxygenase inhibitor that irreversibly acetylates the cyclo-oxygenase enzyme and this results in both a decrease in prostacyclin and thromboxane synthesis. Platelets lack the molecular machinery to re-synthesize cyclo-oxygenase unlike vascular endothelium, hence vascular endothelium-derived prostacyclin is available as an inhibitor of platelet adhesion.

Very large trials such as the International Stroke Trial and the Chinese Acute Stroke Trial attest the value of the early use of aspirin within the first 48 hours of onset of the symptoms of ischaemic stroke. However, the Chinese Acute Stroke Trial did demonstrate a small risk of severe or fatal haemorrhage with the early use of aspirin.

Many studies have been performed which demonstrate the efficacy of aspirin in the long-term secondary prevention of stroke and most studies have demonstrated that low doses of aspirin appear to be as effective as higher dose regimes. The Swedish Aspirin Low-dose Trial (SALT) examined the effect of low dose aspirin (75 mg per day) versus placebo in 1360 patients with TIA, minor stroke or retinal artery occlusion. This demonstrated a statistically significant 8% reduction in risk of stroke or death. A further trial, the Dutch TIA trial study group evaluated the efficacy of Aspirin 30 mg per day versus 283 mg per day in 3131 patients with minor stroke or TIA. This demonstrated that aspirin 30 mg daily was as effective as 283 mg daily in preventing vascular events in minor stroke or TIA. There was also a lower incidence of gastric discomfort and gastric bleeding in the low-dose aspirin group. A very recent meta-analysis, the Antithrombotic Trialist's Collaboration, included 287 studies of antiplatelet therapies which covered 135,000 patients. The end-points were:

- non-fatal myocardial infarction
- non-fatal stroke
- vascular death.

> Low doses of aspirin (75–100 mg/day) seem to be as effective as higher doses in the long-term secondary prevention of stroke

The study found that an absolute reduction of risk of 36 per 1000 in those with previous stroke or TIA was obtained in those receiving antiplatelet therapy over two years. This study again confirmed that lower doses of aspirin (75–150 mg/day) were at least as effective as higher daily doses, however they also concluded that the effects of doses less than 75 mg daily were less certain.

The suggestion that aspirin in low doses of 75 mg should be used in all patients may over simplify the situation. One study in the USA has suggested that some patients require upward adjustment of their aspirin dose to maintain 'an *in vitro* antiplatelet effect'. Further work is required in the area of apparent 'failure' of aspirin therapy as this can, and does, occur. Aspirin failure can sometimes be attributed to non-compliance, however, there is some evidence that concurrent ibuprofen use can interfere with the action of aspirin. In the future, it may be possible to predict those who may be 'aspirin non-responders'.

The most common serious adverse effect of aspirin therapy is gastrointestinal haemorrhage. Initial studies suggested that the incidence of gastrointestinal haemorrhage may be dose related; however, a recent meta-analysis has shown by meta-regression that the incidence of actual gastrointestinal haemorrhage may be independent of the dose of aspirin used. This paper also concluded that the use of modified release preparations of aspirin had no significant effect on the incidence of gastro-intestinal haemorrhage. Factors known to promote gastrointestinal bleeding in patients taking antiplatelet drugs include concurrent use

of non-steroidal anti-inflammatory drugs (NSAIDs) and *Helicobacter pylori* infestation of the stomach. The concurrent use of NSAIDs with aspirin should be avoided if possible and patients may benefit from *H. pylori* eradication if found to have evidence of infection.

> Gastrointestinal haemorrhage is the most common serious adverse effect of aspirin therapy

Combinations of antiplatelet agents have been studied. Dipyridamole is a pyrimidopyrimidine derivative with antiplatelet and vasodilatating properties. Its precise mechanism of antiplatelet action is controversial. Early studies of aspirin and dipyridamole showed no apparent additional benefit in stroke patients. There are many potential reasons for this including under powered studies and the use of short-acting dipyridamole which may give a transient antiplatelet effect. However, the more recent second European Stroke Prevention Study (ESPS2) showed that the use of modified release dipyridamole in doses of 200 mg twice daily did confer additional benefits in terms of secondary stroke prevention and did not appear to significantly increase the risks of major bleeding events. The early trials of dipyridamole were thought to have shown no significant benefit due to the lower doses of standard release dipyridamole used and that the modified release preparations appear to have better bioavailability. The use of modified release dipyridamole 200 mg twice daily is advocated in combination with low-dose aspirin.

> Modified release dipyridamole 200 mg b.i.d. is advocated in combination with low-dose aspirin in the secondary prevention of stroke

Clopidogrel and ticlopidine are newer antiplatelet agents structurally related to thienopyridines. They selectively inhibit adenosine diphosphate-induced platelet aggregation and they do not effect arachidonic acid synthesis. Ticlopidine was successfully shown to reduce stroke, myocardial infarction (MI) and vascular deaths, and evidence exists to show ticlopidine confers greater risk reduction for stroke or death than aspirin and the incidence of gastrointestinal side-effects are significantly less than with aspirin. However, the incidence of neutropaenia associated with ticlopidine has prevented its routine use in the UK.

Clopidogrel is structurally related to ticlopidine. The recent large clopidogrel versus aspirin in patients at risk of ischaemic events (CAPRIE) study directly compared aspirin 325 mg per day with clopidogrel 75 mg per day. The CAPRIE study included patients who had suffered a previous stroke, MI or symptomatic peripheral arterial disease. For the stroke sub-group, the CAPRIE trial failed to demonstrate a significant advantage of clopidogrel over aspirin. The CAPRIE study did demonstrate a significantly lower incidence of gastrointestinal haemorrhage in patients receiving clopidogrel. One must also note that the dose of aspirin employed was relatively high and that the excess risk of bleeding with aspirin could at least in part be accounted for by this.

Trials of other combination anti-platelet agents are planned or are currently being undertaken in patients with cerebrovascular disease. Combinations of aspirin and clopidogrel are currently being assessed in stroke patients and the results are awaited with interest.

Other anti-platelet agents are also currently being studied. Glycoprotein IIb/IIIa receptor antagonists such as abciximab have been used in the acute phase of stroke. Further studies are expected.

Anticoagulation agents

Warfarin and other coumarins act by inhibiting the super-carboxylation process of certain clotting factors in the clotting cascade (II, VII, IX and X). They do this by inhibition of the enzyme vitamin-k epoxide reductase. The dose of warfarin required in any individual is difficult to predict and hence dose monitoring is required, guided by the International Normalized Ratio (INR).

> Warfarin is an anticoagulation agent; it inhibits the super-carboxylation process of clotting factors by inhibiting vitamin-k epoxide reductase

The use of warfarin in atrial fibrillation (AF) has been extensively studied. In western populations, the cause of AF is far more commonly non-valvular heart disease than rheumatic or other valvular disease. The prevalence of non-valvular AF increases with age from 0.5% at age 50–59 to approximately 9% at 80–89 years. Stroke in AF is largely attributable to atrial thrombosis and the risk of stroke is increased five-fold over patients with sinus rhythm. In addition to this, stroke in patients with atrial fibrillation is also associated with a higher mortality than those in sinus rhythm. There appears to be no difference in the risk of stroke in non-valvular AF between males and females or between continuous or paroxysmal atrial fibrillation.

A pooled analysis of five trials of warfarin prophylaxis showed relative risk reduction for stroke of 68% (95 CI 50–79%), and whilst the five trials used various anticoagulant targets (INR between 1.5 and 4.5), the INR range 2–3 conferred the lowest risk of stroke. The incidence of cerebral haemorrhage appears to be 0.1% in controls going up to 0.3% for those receiving warfarin. The greatest risk of intracerebral haemorrhage appears to be associated with uncontrolled hypertension and an INR >3.0. A recent meta-analysis of trials of antithrombotic therapy to prevent stroke in patients with AF concluded that warfarin is substantially more efficacious than aspirin in patients with AF and that these benefits are not offset by the occurrence of major haemorrhage. Lower-intensity warfarin therapy (INR 1.5–2.5) plus aspirin has been compared to standard-intensity warfarin in high-risk patients in the SPAF-3 trial and this demonstrated that standard-intensity warfarin was more effective than low-intensity warfarin plus aspirin. The use of aspirin in combination with low-intensity warfarin protocols can, therefore, not be routinely justified.

> Warfarin is more efficacious than aspirin in preventing stroke in patients with atrial fibrillation

Warfarin substantially reduces the risk of further ischaemic stroke in those patients with previous stroke and non-valvular atrial fibrillation. In the European Atrial Fibrillation Trial (EAFT), patients with non-valvular atrial fibrillation and a recent TIA or minor ischaemic stroke were randomized to open anticoagulation or placebo or double-blind treatment with either 300 mg aspirin daily or placebo. Anticoagulation with warfarin was significantly more effective. The incidence of major bleeding events in the study was 2.8% per year on warfarin and 0.9% on aspirin, although the risks of haemorrhage did not offset the benefits of stroke prevention. In other studies of primary prevention in non-valvular atrial fibrillation, aspirin has been shown to be less effective than warfarin. The target INR range for patients with AF has been extensively debated and in general a target range of 2–3 for the INR gives satisfactory protection whilst minimizing risks of major haemorrhage.

In AF associated with rheumatic valvular disease there is an 18-fold increase in the incidence of ischaemic stroke. In rheumatic mitral valve disease prophylaxis with warfarin can be advised in both primary and secondary prevention. The evidence for this is available by extrapolation from trials in non-valvular atrial fibrillation and expert committee opinion.

> There is an 18-fold increased incidence of ischaemic stroke in patients who have atrial fibrillation and rheumatic valvular disease

The incidence of severe haemorrhagic complications of anticoagulation varies widely in different studies due to different definitions used. The major determinants of haemorrhagic complications are the intensity of anticoagulation used, the length of therapy and the base-line characteristics of the patient. Older patients are proposed to be at higher risk of anticoagulation-related bleeding. However, it is this group who have been shown to receive most benefit. Some studies even refute the claim that older patients are at higher risks of bleeding complications if the INR is closely monitored.

> Older patients receive the most benefit from anticoagulation therapy; however, they are also at the highest risk of related bleeding events

Other specific sub-groups of patients who may benefit specifically from warfarin therapy include those with cardiomyopathy and biological heart valves. Evidence that these patients may benefit from formal anticoagulation is not based on large randomized controlled trials and no large trials looking at these relatively small patient sub-groups have yet been performed.

Evidence supporting the use of warfarin for the secondary prevention of stroke is well established in patients with AF but until recently there was insufficient evidence to suggest that the use of warfarin in patients with sinus rhythm was a safe or effective treatment in the secondary prevention of stroke except where other risk factors co-exist. The Warfarin–Aspirin Recurrent Stroke Study has recently been published. It compared the effects of warfarin (INR 1.4–2.8) and aspirin (325 mg per day) in patients with prior non-cardioembolic stroke. The authors of this study concluded that there is no significant difference between aspirin and warfarin in the prevention of recurrent ischaemic stroke or death in patients with non-cardioembolic stroke, although the incidence of major haemorrhage was 2.22 per 100 patient years in the warfarin group and 1.49 per 100 patient years in the aspirin group. It seems that warfarin could be used in those patients with sinus rhythm where aspirin is unsuitable. However, in view of the alternative antiplatelet agents which have now become available, the number of patients who require warfarin therapy as an alternative to aspirin without co-existent indications for warfarin would appear to be limited.

Antihypertensive agents

Hypertension together with increased age is a major risk factor for stroke and may be the most important risk factor of all. There is a proportionate rise in the incidence of stroke with increasing blood pressure and both systolic and diastolic hypertension is important. A variety of antihypertensive agents are now available including:

- beta-blockers
- alpha-blockers
- diuretics
- calcium channel antagonists
- angiotensin-converting enzyme (ACE) inhibitors
- angiotensin II antagonists
- centrally acting agents, such as methyldopa and hydralazine.

A variety of trials have examined the efficacy of these agents both as single- and multi-drug regimes.

> Hypertension is the most important treatable risk factor for stroke

A clear body of evidence has emerged to support the use of antihypertensive medications in the prevention of stroke, although the vast majority of antihypertensive trials have focused on the primary prevention of stroke. A meta-analysis of trials of antihypertensive agents used in the treatment of patients who had already suffered stroke did, however, conclude that benefit can be

demonstrated with the use of antihypertensive medications in the secondary prevention of stroke. Current available data does not allow verification as to whether the benefits observed were dependent on initial blood pressure level or not.

Simple agents such as diuretics may be the most effective antihypertensive medications available. One Chinese study compared the diuretic indapamide with placebo and even though only a modest average reduction in blood pressure of 5/2 mmHg was achieved (lowering the average to 144/87 mmHg), this resulted in a 29% relative risk reduction in fatal or non-fatal stroke. The Swedish Trial in Old Patients with hypertension (STOP-hypertension) further demonstrated that the use of a beta-blocker or diuretic could prevent 73 strokes per 1000 patients treated for five years. Further evidence as to the preferred choice of anti-hypertensive agent was then provided by the Medical Research Council (MRC) trial of hypertension in older patients, which compared the use of the beta-blocker atenolol and the diuretic combination hydrochlorthiazide and amiloride and found that diuretics were superior to beta-blockers. Many trials of anti-hypertensive agents have been shown to confer benefits in terms of primary stroke prevention, see Figure 8.2.

> Modest reductions in blood pressure can translate in to large drops in stroke risk, eg lowering blood pressure by 5/2 mmHg lead to a 29% stroke-risk reduction in one Chinese study

Even modest reductions in blood pressure have been shown to translate into substantial reductions in the risk of stroke. The Hypertension Optimal Treatment (HOT) study showed that treating hypertension to a target blood pressure of 140/85 mmHg achieved a greater benefit in terms of reduction in the incidence of stroke, although this target generally required a multi-drug regime and a concerted effort on behalf of the physician and patient. Good blood pressure control has also been shown to be particularly effective in diabetic patients and this patient

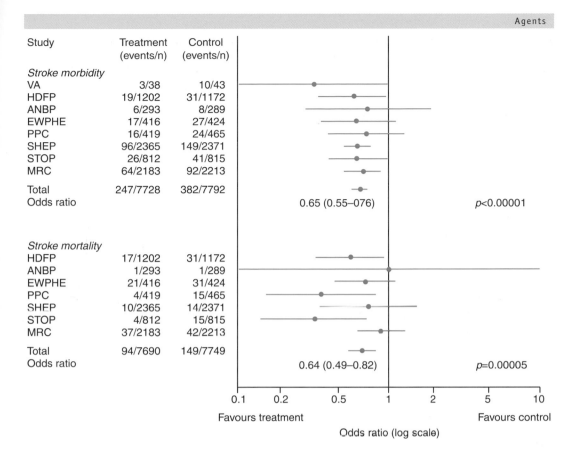

Study	Treatment (events/n)	Control (events/n)
Stroke morbidity		
VA	3/38	10/43
HDFP	19/1202	31/1172
ANBP	6/293	8/289
EWPHE	17/416	27/424
PPC	16/419	24/465
SHEP	96/2365	149/2371
STOP	26/812	41/815
MRC	64/2183	92/2213
Total	247/7728	382/7792
Odds ratio		0.65 (0.55–076) p<0.00001
Stroke mortality		
HDFP	17/1202	31/1172
ANBP	1/293	1/289
EWPHE	21/416	31/424
PPC	4/419	15/465
SHEP	10/2365	14/2371
STOP	4/812	15/815
MRC	37/2183	42/2213
Total	94/7690	149/7749
Odds ratio		0.64 (0.49–0.82) p=0.00005

Favours treatment   Favours control

Odds ratio (log scale)

Figure 8.2

Results of meta-analysis of stroke morbidity and mortality end-points in selected hypertension trials. Left, absolute numbers; Right, odds ratios and 95% confidence intervals.

ANBP, Australian National Blood Pressure Study; EWPHE, European Working Party on High Blood Pressure in the Elderly; HDFP, Hypertension Detection and Follow-up Program; MRC, Medical Research Council; PPC, Practice in Primary Care; SHEP, Systolic Hypertension in the Elderly; STOP, Swedish Trial in Old Patients with Hypertension; VA, Veterans Administration Cooperative Study on Antihypertensive Agents.

Adapted with permission from from Insua JT *et al*. Drug treatment of hypertension in the elderly: a meta-analysis. *Ann Intern Med* 1994; **121**: 355–62

group in particular should make a concerted effort to reach a normotensive state.

Antihypertensive regimens are not without adverse effects. Antihypertensive medications have an associated risk of postural hypotension, particularly in the elderly and clearly this results in risks, such as:

* hip and colles fracture
* loss of confidence
* loss of independence.

Other adverse effects of antihypertensive medications have been proposed but as yet they are not established; an increased risk of gastrointestinal bleeding with calcium antagonists has been proposed although this relationship has not been substantiated. Recent concern has also been raised about a potential relationship between long-term antihypertensive use and cancer, but again no relationship has been proven at the present time. In general antihypertensive drugs are well-tolerated.

Angiotensin-converting enzyme inhibitors

Angiotensin-converting enzyme (ACE) inhibitors work by inhibiting the action of the serum enzyme ACE, which promotes the conversion of the hormone angiotensin I to angiotensin II. Angiotensin II is a potent vasoconstrictor and also acts at the adrenal medulla, increasing secretion of aldosterone with subsequent sodium retention. This is a simplified overview of the role of ACE in the pathogenesis of cardio- and cerebrovascular disease and ACE inhibitors have other far-reaching beneficial effects:

- they improve endothelial function
- they alter collagen disposition in vessel walls.

Angiotensin-converting enzyme inhibitors are effective antihypertensive agents, however, it appears that their beneficial effects may not be entirely related to their hypotensive actions. Indeed, the Study to Evaluate Carotid Ultrasound changes in patients treated with Ramipril and vitamin E (SECURE) demonstrated that the progression of atherosclerosis was significantly reduced by ramipril compared to placebo.

> ACE inhibitors have many affects which help in stroke prevention: they lower blood pressure, improve endothelial function and alter collagen disposition in blood vessel walls

Other more recent studies have looked at the effects of ACE inhibitors using 'hard end-points', such as stroke, MI and vascular death. The Heart Outcome Protection Study (HOPE) was a large randomized controlled trial which included patients with previous stroke but also included those with other vascular disease such as ischaemic heart disease. The study was not specifically powered to look at the effects of ACE inhibitors in stroke patients. The HOPE study recruited over 9000 patients and compared the ACE inhibitor ramipril with either vitamin E or placebo. The follow-up period was 4–6 years. The magnitude of blood pressure reduction was modest (3.8 mmHg systolic and 2.8 mmHg diastolic) although the relative risk reduction of

any stroke was 32% in the ramipril group compared to placebo. The relative risk of fatal stroke was reduced by 61%. Clearly the relative risk reduction appears disproportionate to the relatively modest reduction in blood pressure and may be accounted for, in part, by the other beneficial effect of ACE inhibitors. Figure 8.3 shows the Kaplan-Meier analysis of ramipril and placebo for stroke in the HOPE study.

The HOPE study was not specifically powered to look at the secondary prevention of stroke and indeed the number of patients with previous stroke in the study was relatively small. The more recent Perindopril Prevention Against Recurrent Stroke Study (PROGRESS) was specifically powered to examine the efficacy of an ACE inhibitor-based antihypertensive regime in stroke patients. Patients were randomized to receive either the ACE inhibitor perindopril plus the thiazide diuretic indapamide or to placebo. Outcomes included recurrent stroke, disability, cognitive decline and major vascular events. The study identified similar adherence to therapy in both placebo and active treatment groups. There was a 28% (CI 17–38%) risk reduction of stroke and a 26% (CI 16–33%) risk reduction in major vascular death (defined as vascular death, non-fatal MI or non-fatal stroke) in the active treatment group compared to placebo. One stroke was prevented in every 23 patients treated for five years. One major vascular event was prevented for every 18 patients treated for five years. Even greater benefit was seen for patients in Asia, patients who sustained haemorrhagic stroke and those treated with the combination of perindopril and indapamide. A reduction in the incidence of stroke, MI, disability and cognitive decline was proven in the PROGRESS study in those on active treatment compared to placebo. Interestingly PROGRESS also demonstrated that benefit was obtained by patients across the whole spectrum of entry blood pressure, including those with normal blood pressure.

PROGRESS also examined the effects of a perindopril-based antihypertensive regime on the incidence of major vascular events including

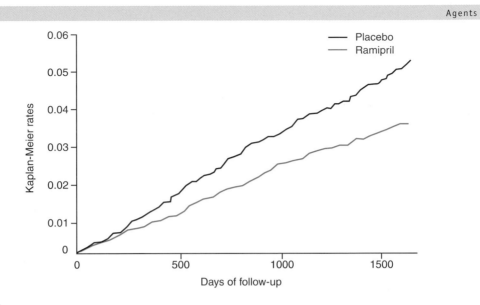

Figure 8.3
Reduction in stroke among those high-risk patients treated with either ramipril or placebo in the HOPE study.

Reprinted from Bosch *et al*. *BMJ* 2002; **324**: 699–702 with permission from the BMJ Publishing Group

vascular death and non-fatal MI and again a significant benefit was obtained. Similar rates of withdrawal from both active treatment and placebo were seen; however in the active treatment group withdrawal from treatment was more frequent due to hypotension (1%) and cough (1.7%). There were 0.7% fewer withdrawals due to heart failure.

It must be noted that the greatest benefit in the PROGRESS trial was seen in patients treated with the combination therapy of perindopril and indapamide. Patients treated with this combination had blood pressure lowered by a mean of 12/5 mmHg. Patients on perindopril alone had their blood pressure lowered by a mean of only 5/3 mmHg. Stroke risk was not discernibly different between participants who received perindopril alone and single placebo, although the trial protocol was not designed to assess the effect of the use of indapamide as a single agent. Figure 8.4 demonstrates the comparison between active treatment and placebo.

Angiotensin II antagonists

The beneficial effects of the use of angiotensin II antagonists in the primary prevention of stroke has recently been demonstrated in the LIFE study. Patients were selected for this particular study on the basis of evidence of left ventricular hypertrophy (LVH) identified on ECG. The study demonstrated that losartan, when used in hypertensive patients, appeared to reduce the incidence of stroke when compared to atenolol (even though the mean reduction of blood pressure was identical between the two study arms). This would suggest that other beneficial properties may be available from the use of losartan other than its antihypertensive effect. Whether this is the case in the secondary prevention of stroke and whether this is likely to be a 'class-effect' shared by all angiotensin II antagonists is still to be proven. Figure 8.5 shows the reduction in rate of stroke comparing the beta-blocker atenolol and the angiotensin antagonist losartan.

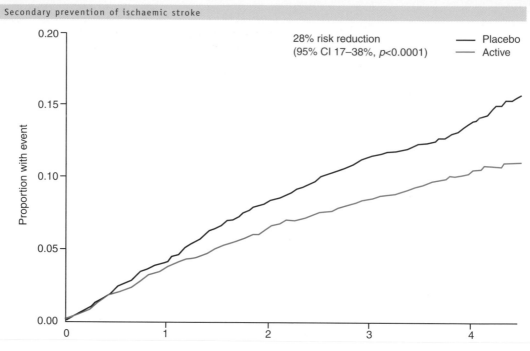

Figure 8.4
Reduction in stroke among those stroke patients treated with active therapy (perindopril with or without indapamide) in the PROGRESS study.

Reprinted with permission from Elsevier, PROGRESS Collaborative Group. *Lancet* 2001; **358**: 1033–41

> The angiotensin II antagonist losartan has been shown to reduce the incidence of stroke when compared to atenolol (a beta-blocker), but both drugs achieved similar blood pressure reductions

Lipid-lowering agents

There is a clear relationship between serum lipids and atherosclerosis, although it has taken some time to establish a clear relationship between modifying the serum lipid profile and decreasing the risk of stroke. Abnormalities of cholesterol, triglycerides, low-density lipoprotein (LDL) and high-density lipoproteins (HDL) are regarded as atherosclerotic risk factors, and the progression and degree of carotid atherosclerosis are directly related to cholesterol and LDL and inversely related to HDL. A number of lipid-lowering agents exist including:

- cholesterol transport inhibitors (ezetimibe)
- HMG-CoA reductase inhibitors (statins)
- fibrates
- cholesterol binding agents (eg cholestyramine)
- omega fish oils.

Each of these agents has a specific propensity to reduce either cholesterol or triglycerides and some agents have a beneficial effect on all lipid parameters. Some other novel agents should become available in the near future.

The pathogenesis of stroke is multi-factorial and can be one of multiple sub-types, not all of which can be attributed to atherosclerosis.

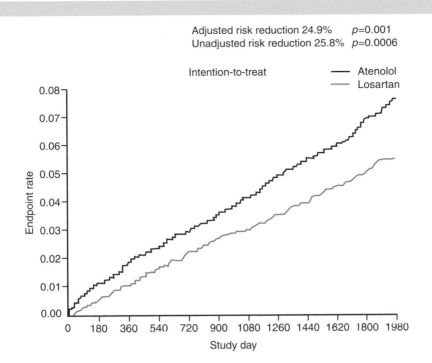

Adjusted risk reduction 24.9%   *p*=0.001
Unadjusted risk reduction 25.8%   *p*=0.0006

Figure 8.5
Reduction of stroke end-point in LIFE study. Comparable blood pressure reduction with losartan was associated with lower stroke rate than atenolol.

Reprinted with permission from Elsevier, Dahlof B *et al. Lancet* 2002; **359**: 995–1003

This may be one of the reasons why a consistent significant relationship between cholesterol reduction and stroke has been difficult to establish. Both primary and secondary prevention trials of HMG-CoA reductase inhibitors have demonstrated a substantial reduction in ischaemic stroke and MI in those receiving active treatment. Various meta-analyses have been performed which support this. The Cholesterol and Recurrent Events (CARE) trial also demonstrated that amongst patients with previous MI whose cholesterol levels are average, pravastatin significantly reduced the incidence of stroke and TIA. In the Long-term Intervention with Pravastatin in Ischaemic Disease (LIPID) trial pravastatin reduced the risk of sustaining stroke of any cause in those who had suffered previous MI or unstable angina. Interestingly, an inverse

relationship has previously been suggested between total cholesterol and haemorrhagic stroke.

> Lipid-lowering agents help to reduce atherosclerosis and thereby prevent some atherosclerosis-related forms of stroke, eg ischaemic stroke

More recently the Heart Protection Study (HPS) enrolled over 20,500 subjects and was a prospective, double-blind, randomized controlled trial with a 2x2 factorial design investigating prolonged use (>5 years) of simvastatin 40 mg and a cocktail of antioxidant vitamins (vitamin E, vitamin C and beta-carotene). The study specifically included patients with a high risk of coronary heart disease (CHD). The definition of 'high risk' included patients with a previous TIA or stroke (with a minimum total cholesterol [TC] ≥3.5 mmol/L at entry). Treatment with simvastatin 40 mg was associated with benefit across all patient groups regardless of age, gender or baseline cholesterol value and it proved to be safe and well tolerated. There was a:

- 12% reduction in total mortality
- 17% reduction in vascular mortality
- 24% reduction in CHD events
- 27% reduction in all strokes
- 16% reduction in non-coronary revascularizations.

> Simvastatin has been shown to reduce vascular mortality, CHD events, strokes and non-coronary revascularizations in all patients regardless of their gender, age or baseline cholesterol level

Preliminary results of the HPS were negative for the antioxidant vitamin cocktail studied. This landmark trial demonstrated a significant advantage of using simvastatin 40 mg in patients with previous stroke or TIA in preventing further stroke and death. A striking

feature of this study was that even patients with relatively low serum cholesterol (TC ≥3.5 mmol/L) still attained benefit from a statin, the magnitude of reduction in the relative risk of stroke also appeared to be very impressive. Figure 8.6 demonstrates the reduction of ischaemic stroke in the heart protection study.

Reduction of serum cholesterol and modification of the LDL/HDL profile is currently recommended in the presence of CHD, but whether any absolute benefit is conferred in the secondary prevention of stroke in the absence of co-existing coronary artery disease is still to be proven in a large randomized controlled trial of stroke patients. The Stroke Prevention by Aggressive Reduction of Cholesterol Levels (SPARCL) study is a large multi-centre randomized controlled trial of the HMG-CoA reductase inhibitor atorvastatin versus placebo. It is specifically looking at those patients with a past history of cerebrovascular disease with an absence of overt CHD. The planned follow-up is three years and the results are currently awaited.

The safety profile of statins is good with relatively few patients in the trials withdrawing from treatment due to side-effects. Hepatic,

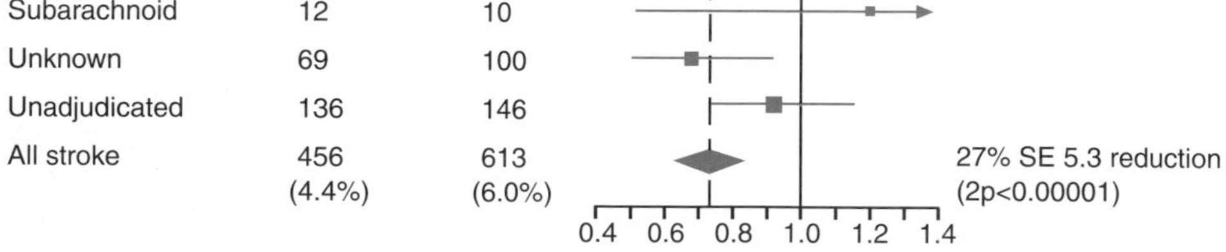

Simvastatin:Stroke by aetiology

Stroke aetiology	Statin (10,269)	Placebo (10,267)	Risk ratio and 95% CI Statin better Statin worse
Ischaemic	242	376	
Haemorrhagic	45	53	
Subarachnoid	12	10	
Unknown	69	100	
Unadjudicated	136	146	
All stroke	456 (4.4%)	613 (6.0%)	27% SE 5.3 reduction (2p<0.00001)

Figure 8.6
Reduction of ischaemic stroke in the Heart Protection Study.

CI, confidence interval

Reprinted with permission from Elsevier, Heart Protection Study Collaborative Group. *Lancet* 2002; **630**: 7–22 musculoskeletal and renal systems can be adversely affected – some of these side-effects can be severe, although their occurrence is uncommon. Headache and nausea are other less serious side-effects of statins although they do not commonly result in withdrawal from therapy.

> Although lipid-lowering using statins is relatively safe, in rare cases serious problems can affect the renal, hepatic and musculoskeletal systems

Insulin and oral anti-diabetic agents

Diabetics require special consideration. Good evidence exists that the use of insulin regimes in type I diabetes mellitus and oral hypoglycaemic agents with or without the addition of insulin in type II diabetes reduces the incidence of microvascular complications. The incidence of retinopathy, neuropathy and nephropathy is lower in patients with tight glycaemic control. Unfortunately there is little evidence to demonstrate a definite relationship between the incidence of macrovascular disease, such as stroke, and glycaemic control. The practice of maintaining long-term normoglycaemia is clearly justified by the reduction of microvascular complications. However, one can not state categorically that tight glycaemic control will reduce an individual's propensity to stroke.

Identifying diabetes in any patient presenting with stroke or TIA is particularly important as they will benefit from modification of risk factors. The importance of reducing other risks, eg smoking, hypertension and dyslipidaemia, in diabetic patients cannot be overemphasized.

> There is currently little evidence to link stroke reduction with tight glycaemic control; however, stroke patients who are diabetic will benefit enormously by reducing other stroke risk factors

Evidence is beginning to emerge that in patients with impaired glucose tolerance, progression to type II diabetes can be prevented by lifestyle changes, probably by the use of the biguinide metformin, and potentially by other drugs. Metformin has also recently been shown to potentially reduce the risk of macrovascular disease. Unlike sulphonylureas, the use of metformin is becoming more widespread due to these beneficial effects.

The glitazones group of drugs holds out some promise and study results are awaited.

Aids to smoking cessation

The smoking of cigarettes is a significant independent risk factor for stroke. The benefit obtained through smoking cessation in one study of male smokers was dependent on the amount of tobacco previously smoked. People who smoke less than 20 cigarettes daily revert to the risk level of those who had never smoked whilst those who previously smoked more heavily still maintained a greater than two-fold risk compared to those who had never smoked. These benefits were seen within five years of the last cigarette smoked. The greatest benefit obtained from smoking cessation is seen in those who are also hypertensive.

> Stroke risk of smokers can return to that of a non-smoker within five years of quitting cigarettes

Effective aids to smoking cessation are nicotine replacement therapies and the anti-depressant related medication bupropion. Nicotine replacement therapy in studies has not unduly affected cardiovascular risk. In one study of bupropion versus placebo the rate of withdrawal from therapy due to side-effects was 8% versus 5%, respectively. The drug seems to be well tolerated. There have been occasional case reports of serious adverse reactions including seizures, myocardial ischaemia and hypersensitivity reactions, although these appear to be uncommon. No specific studies have identified the risks and benefits in the secondary prevention of stroke with the use of bupropion.

Procedures

Carotid endarterectomy

Carotid endarterectomy (CEA) is the procedure of physically removing carotid atheroma. In the UK current indications for carotid endarterectomy are those patients who have recently experienced a TIA or non-disabling stroke who are found to have an ipsilateral stenosis of the internal or common carotid circulation of 70–99%. The degree of carotid stenosis can be estimated by a number of methods including:

- Doppler ultrasound
- magnetic resonance arteriography
- invasive carotid angiography.

In the UK carotid endarterectomy is indicated for patients who have had a TIA or non-disabling stroke and also have ipsilateral stenosis (70–99%) of the internal or common carotid circulation

The European Carotid Surgery Trial (ECST) and the North American Symptomatic Carotid Endarterectomy Trial (NASCET) used different techniques to estimate the degree of carotid stenosis. The NASCET method may have underestimated the degree of stenosis, although the trial illustrated that CEA, when performed by a skilled surgeon, may confer significant reduction in further stroke. Figure 8.7 demonstrates results obtained from the NASCET trial.

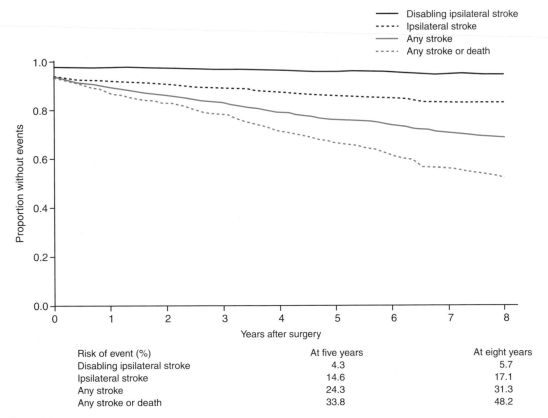

Risk of event (%)	At five years	At eight years
Disabling ipsilateral stroke	4.3	5.7
Ipsilateral stroke	14.6	17.1
Any stroke	24.3	31.3
Any stroke or death	33.8	48.2

Figure 8.7
Long-term results of carotid endarterectomy in the NASCET trial.

Reproduced with permission from Ferguson *et al. Stroke* 1999; **30**: 1751–8

The technique of CEA has been refined and may now be performed with regional anaesthesia. The rate of peri-operative stroke, the main direct surgical risk of the procedure, has decreased and there may be moves in the future to expand the indications for surgery for stenosis to less than 70%.

Cartotid angioplasty and stenting

Carotid endarterectomy has been shown to be an effective form of treatment in selected patients; evidence is becoming available that carotid angioplasty and stent insertion (CAS) is a safe and effective alternative to an open surgical procedure. Several randomized trials are currently underway, the long-term results of which are awaited.

The technique employs the use of an angioplasty balloon and stent insertion. However, due to the potentially catastrophic risks of embolizing an atheromatous plaque, various cerebral protection devices are being developed. Balloon inflation, retractable filter baskets and methods of flow reversal appear to be effective methods of reducing the risks of peri-procedural stroke.

Patients who may be particularly suitable for CAS include those with previous carotid endarterectomy and re-stenosis, post-radiotherapy carotid stenosis and those with a high surgical risk for CEA, eg those with significant cardiopulmonary disease. In addition to these groups, those patients with plaques inaccessible to an open surgical procedure (eg a plaque extending into the internal carotid system as it enters the skull base) may be particularly suitable for CAS.

As more experience is gained with CAS and long-term observations become available this technique may become well practiced and this could prove to be a valuable tool in secondary stroke prevention.

Further reading

A randomised, blinded, trial of clopidogrel versus aspirin in patients at risk of ischaemic events (CAPRIE). CAPRIE Steering Committee. *Lancet* 1996; **348**: 1329–39.

Beneficial effect of carotid endarterectomy in symptomatic patients with high-grade carotid stenosis. North American Symptomatic Carotid Endarterectomy Trial Collaborators. *N Engl J Med* 1991; **325**: 445–53.

Bosch J, Yusuf S, Pogue J et al. Use of ramipril in preventing stroke: double blind randomised trial. *BMJ* 2002; **324**: 699–702.

CAVATAS investigators. Endovascular versus surgical treatment in patients with carotid stenosis in the Carotid and Vertebral Artery Transluminal Angioplasty study (CAVATAS): randomised trial. *Lancet* 2001; **357**: 1729–37.

Collaborative meta-analysis of randomised trials of antiplatelet therapy for prevention of death, myocardial infarction, and stroke in high risk patients. *BMJ* 2002; **324**: 71–86.

Dahlof B, Devereux RB, Kjeldsen SE et al. Cardiovascular morbidity and mortality in the Losartan Intervention For Endpoint reduction in hypertension study (LIFE): a randomised trial against atenolol. *Lancet* 2002; **359**: 995–1003.

Diener HC, Cunha L, Forbes C et al. European Stroke Prevention Study. 2. Dipyridamole and acetylsalicylic acid in the secondary prevention of stroke. *J Neurol Sci* 1996; **143**: 1–13.

MRC/BHF Heart Protection Study of cholesterol lowering with simvastatin in 20,536 high-risk individuals: a randomised placebo-controlled trial. *Lancet* 2002; **360**: 7–22.

MRC European Carotid Surgery Trial: interim results for symptomatic patients with severe (70-99%) or with mild (0-29%) carotid stenosis. European Carotid Surgery Trialists' Collaborative Group. *Lancet* 1991; **337**: 1235–43.

PROGRESS Collaborative Group: Randomised trial of a perindopril-based blood-pressure-lowering regimen among 6105 individuals with previous stroke or transient ischaemic attack. *Lancet* 2001; **358**: 1033–41.

Secondary prevention in non-rheumatic atrial fibrillation after transient ischaemic attack or minor stroke. EAFT (European Atrial Fibrillation Trial) Study Group. *Lancet* 1993; **342**: 1255–62.

9. Complications and avoiding complications

Immobility
Falls
Infection
Nutrition
Psychological morbidity
Central nervouse system dysfunction
Pain after stroke
Complications of treatment

Table 9.1
Some important complications after acute stroke

General medical complications
- dehydration or volume depletion
- malnutrition
- thromboembolism
  - deep vein thrombosis (DVT)
  - pulmonary embolism (PTE)
- infection
- urinary tract infection (UTI)
- chest infection
- adverse dug reaction (ADR)

Central nervous system complications
- recurrent stroke
- cerebral oedema
- increased pressure
- haemorrhagic transformation of infarction
- depressed mood
- emotional lability
- shoulder pain
- shoulder–hand syndrome (ie reflex sympathetic dystrophy)
- cold limb
- central post-stroke pain (thalamic syndrome)
- spasticity
- post-stroke seizures

Complications following stroke may occur as a consequence of the stroke or as a result of various treatments instituted after stroke. Table 9.1 outlines common complications.

Immobility

Immobility is a common feature after stroke, particularly in the days following the event. Complications following immobility may be eminently preventable.

Deep vein thrombosis and pulmonary thromboembolism

Venous thromboembolic disease is a potentially fatal complication of immobility with pulmonary embolus accounting for up to 25% of early deaths following acute stroke. Immobility of any cause is an acknowledged risk factor for venous thromboembolic disease. Patients with stroke are frequently not administered thrombo-prophylaxis and this offers an opportunity to intervene and reduce morbidity and mortality. Two out of every three cases of venous thromboembolic disease may be preventable if thrombo-prophylaxis was used when indicated.

Studies suggest that the use of subcutaneous low molecular weight heparins are more effective than unfractionated heparin in the prevention of thromboembolic disease. The use of thromboembolic prevention stockings is, however, favoured by some as there is a perceived slightly increased risk of haemorrhagic complication with the use of subcutaneous heparin. The utility of these stockings is subject to an ongoing trial. These stockings should not be used when there is serious arterial insufficiency present in the legs. However, when a DVT is established, support stockings may be beneficial and should help prevent the development of post-thrombotic leg complications. Treatment of established thromboembolic complications would include anticoagulation with heparin or a low molecular weight heparin and warfarin. The situation is more complex when a haemorrhagic stroke has occurred and careful balancing of risks and benefits is required. An inferior vena caval filter may be required as an alternative or in addition to other treatment in selected cases.

> Complications following immobility include skin pressure problems, deep vein thrombosis, pulmonary thromboembolism and osteopaenia

Skin pressure problems

Prolonged periods of immobility result in poor skin perfusion and nutrition at areas in contact with mattresses – this results in the formation of 'pressure sores'. Patients with stroke should be assessed for risk factors associated with pressure sores and the appropriate level of intervention should be employed. The use of special mattresses and automated turning beds has shown particular promise in reducing the incidence of pressure sore formation and improving patient comfort.

Osteopaenia and osteoporosis

Immobility following stroke has been associated with loss of bone mineral density and this may be an important factor in the increased risk of hip fracture seen after stroke. Furthermore, there is evidence that early mobilization after stroke may prevent bone loss and subsequently avoid the propensity to fractures.

Falls

Falls following stroke are a common problem with a reported frequency of 11.5% in one study. The risk of hip fracture in a patient with previous stroke is four-fold that of the background population. Patients who sustain a fracture also have a poorer survival rate. Risk factors most strongly associated with the highest rate of fall include moderate to severe disability as rated on the Barthel Index on admission and dysphasia; particular attention should be paid to these high-risk groups. Approximately 70% of falls occur during the daytime. Underlying medical causes, such as drugs and cardiac arrhythmias, are potentially

treatable aetiologies and falls prevention 'care pathways' which look at environmental factors, functional state of the patient, etc are felt to be an effective means of reducing the incidence of falls.

> A person who has suffered a stroke has a four-fold increased risk of hip fracture associated with a fall

Infection

Infections of the lower-respiratory tract and urinary tract are common following stroke. The incidence of pneumonia is higher when:

- the patient has experienced stroke in multiple locations
- chronic obstructive airways disease co-exists
- aspiration is demonstrated on videofluoroscopy.

Pneumonia occurring in the first six months after stroke is significantly more frequent in those with hypertension, diabetes and poor laryngeal elevation on videofluoroscopy. Aspiration is most commonly associated with multiple strokes, brainstem stroke and stroke involving subcortical structures. Strategies for dealing with these problems generally involve identifying those patients at greatest risk of pneumonia using bedside assessment and/or videofluoroscopy. Once identified, these patients can be given particular attention looking at aspects, such as dietary consistency, the need for percutaneous endoscopic gastrostomy (PEG) feeding, etc in an effort to reduce the incidence of lower respiratory tract infection. This strategy seems to be effective.

Urinary tract infection is a common occurrence following stroke and may occur in up to one-quarter of patients. It is particularly common in those with indwelling urinary catheters. An important strategy is to ensure that urinary catheters are removed at an early opportunity. If a long-term catheter is deemed necessary then specific catheters, such as sialastic devices, should be used. Some doctors even advocate the use of supra-pubic devices to avoid long-term infective complications.

> Up to one-quarter of stroke patients develop a urinary tract infection

Fever and infection early after ischaemic stroke seem to be associated with more severe neurological deficits on admission. Fever occurs more commonly on day one and two than days three to seven following stroke. Up to one-half of infections in early stroke may have been acquired before the stroke.

Nutrition

In the acute phase of stroke the oral route for the administration of fluids, nutrition and medications is frequently unavailable until the swallow reflex is formally assessed. Dehydration and eventually malnutrition supervene – both are associated with a poor outcome from stroke.

> Every effort should be made to maintain adequate hydration and nutrition in stroke patients

Fluid intake in dysphagic stroke patients is frequently inadequate and it is important to ensure that adequate supplementary fluids are prescribed either enterally or parenterally. Thickened drinks are one solution in patients whose swallow is not safe for normal fluid intake, although fluid balance needs to be carefully assessed to ensure adequate hydration.

Enteral feeding

Enteral feeding may be introduced, where the swallow has not sufficiently recovered, by means of naso-gastric feeding tubes or other definitive devices, such as percutaneous endoscopic gastrostomy (PEG) feeding tubes, jejunostomy tubes or an equivalent.

Nasogastric (NG) tube insertion allows a temporary route for feeding in the presence of an intact gut. A major complication of NG tubes is displacement of the tube. This results in the risk of spillage of feed material into the pharynx and subsequent risk of aspiration – if the tube accidentally comes up from the stomach, where it is supposed to be, the liquid feed can be pumped in to the lungs. Coughing and decreased levels of consciousness are risk factors for NG tube displacement. Patients suspected of having displacement of the NG tube should be considered for repeat chest radiographs to confirm the tube is maintained in position.

> Percutaneous endoscopic gastrostomy is a fairly secure route of administering nutrition and medication; however, mild complications can occur in up to 70% of patients

Percutaneous endoscopic gastrostomy is a widely used technique that offers a relatively secure pathway for the administration of nutrition and medications via the enteral route. If swallowing is slow to return to normal, PEG tubes are often inserted to avoid prolonged feeding by the NG route. The method is unfortunately not without risk and 30-day mortality rates have been reported of 4.1–26%. Complications can occur in up to 70% of patients, however, these are usually minor. Predictors of poor outcome after PEG insertion include older age, male gender, diabetes and some specific indications for PEG. Some of these factors could be considered when assessing a patient's suitability for PEG insertion.

Recovery of swallow may still occur after the insertion of PEG tubes and in certain cases long-term follow-up of swallow has enabled patients to resume a normal diet. Removal of the PEG tube will clearly avoid complications of the prosthetic device and will also allow the patient to benefit from other important factors of a normal diet including the social aspects of eating.

Psychological morbidity

Depressed mood

Depressive symptoms following stroke are a common phenomena. A study using the Beck Depression Inventory estimates up to 27% of patients demonstrate symptoms two weeks after stroke. The prevalence of major depression is thought to be lower at approximately 5.6%. Older patients and people with a history of depressive illness appear to be most vulnerable to depression after stroke. Stroke seems to be most closely associated with depression when the lesion involves the left hemisphere or brain stem.

> 27% of patients show depressive symptoms two weeks after their stroke

Depression after stroke is associated with impaired recovery in activities of daily living (ADL) during the first two years after stroke. Improvement in depressive symptoms is associated with improvement in scores for ADL. Some studies suggest that non-pharmacological mechanisms may be important in improvements of ADLs, however, pharmacological agents still have an important role to play in treating post-stroke depression. Appropriate intervention, including the use of pharmacological agents, has been shown to improve mortality following stroke.

The frequency of suicidal ideas has been shown to increase with time elapsed from stroke. Recurrent stroke, depressive symptoms, more disabling stroke and right-sided stroke correlate with suicidal ideas 15 months after stroke. Early identification of these patients and appropriate intervention is clearly indicated. Patients should be routinely screened for depression and anxiety and this should be re-evaluated during rehabilitation. A trial of treatment with antidepressant medication will be indicated if depression is identified.

Anxiety

Anxiety is a common problem after an acute stroke. Situations that provoke anxiety might include fear of falling when transferring or a generalized anxiety disorder not linked to any particular situation may be present. Some people cope with anxiety better than others. Some may cope by avoiding the situation that provokes the feelings. Certain antidepressant drugs (eg paroxetine) can be tried. Patients with depression and anxiety may require evaluation by psychology or psychiatry services.

> Anxiety is common after stroke

Emotionalism

After a stroke crying is not uncommon. An impairment of the control of crying (and more rarely laughing), where it can arise with minimal provocation, is known as emotionalism or emotional lability. When this is severe or disruptive an antidepressant medication may be tried.

Fatigue

Fatigue is a common experience after stroke and has many potential causes, including the effort required to take part in a rehabilitation programme. Fatigue has recently been shown in neurobehavioural studies to be associated with brainstem and thalamic lesions. This may be related to damage to the reticular activating system. Fatigue may be associated with attentional problems and may severely limit the patient's capacity for recovery. Strategies specific to the individual patient may need to be devised to address the problem. Post-stroke fatigue may occur independently from depressive illness.

Cognitive impairment

Certain specific impairments, which can masquerade as cognitive impairment, are sometimes found in stroke patients. These exclude aphasia but include:

- visuospatial neglect
- apraxia
- impaired learning
- reduced attention.

Their importance is that they may explain an otherwise inexplicable disability; for example, impaired attention, planning or visuospatial abilities may explain difficulty in dressing.

Cognitive impairment can be due to a single stroke or be the consequence of multiple strokes and can complicate recovery from stroke.

Social reintegration

Social reintegration is a major factor in the rehabilitation process and impacts on many other aspects of living with disability. The patient's perceptions of their level of both functional and social performance seem to be the key factors in social reintegration.

> Psychological problems that can affect stroke patients include depression, anxiety, emotionalism, fatigue, cognitive impairment and social reintegration issues

Sexual dysfunction following stroke may be as frequent as 58.6% in males and 44% in women. This can be due to either loss of libido or physical sexual dysfunction. Those patients with physical sexual dysfunction have significantly more depressive symptoms and more impaired activities of daily living. Left hemisphere lesions and post-stroke depression appear to be independent predictors of sexual dysfunction after stroke.

> Up to 44% of women and 58.6% of men may experience sexual dysfunction after a stroke

Central nervous system dysfunction
Early complications

Early neurological complications after acute stroke include cerebral oedema, raised intracranial pressure with possible coning and seizures. Cerebral infarctions can become haemorrhagic and this may be symptomatic.

Sleep apnoea

Sleep apnoea may occur in up to 59% of patients with stroke. Patients with sleep apnoea may have a higher incidence of ischaemic heart disease and often suffer earlier cerebral infarction. Sleep apnoea does not seem to be linked to any particular site of stroke but is associated with delirium, depressed mood, latency in reaction in response to verbal stimuli and impaired activities of daily living. At present it is not clear whether treatment of sleep apnoea with positive airways pressure non-invasive ventilation results in reversal of these complications or not.

> Sleep apnoea is linked to delirium, depressed mood and impaired activities of daily living, and up to 59% of stroke patients suffer from it at some point

Urinary dysfunction

Dysfunction of the urinary tract is a common complication following stroke. Urinary retention may occur in as many as 29% of stroke patients. Cognitive impairment, diabetes mellitus, aphasia, poor admission functional status scores and infection seem to be associated factors. Identifying those patients at risk of urinary retention and offering earlier treatment will ultimately reduce morbidity. Urinary incontinence is also a common problem after stroke and in some studies the rate of improvement to continence was only 25%. Patients aged over 75 years have less chance of regaining continence and subjects with lacunar infarction are more likely to regain continence compared to those with anterior circulation infarction. Incontinence three months after stroke is associated with greater rates of institutionalization and worse disability.

A relatively conservative approach to urinary dysfunction is advocated in the first three to six months after stroke as a spontaneous improvement in symptoms is frequently seen during this period.

Spasticity

Spasticity is an involuntary contraction of muscle that is frequently observed after stroke. If left untreated permanent contracture formation may occur and this worsens functional outcomes. The use of limb positioning and splints may be one effective method of preventing complications of spasticity. Antispasticity agents such as baclofen, tizanidine and dantrolene can significantly reduce the handicap of spasticity. Spasticity assessed by the modified Ashworth scoring system, strength testing, functional assessment and pain questionnaire is significantly improved by the use of antispastic agents. Side-effects of treatment can include decreased muscle tone and weakness; however, this can be surprisingly uncommon with agents such as tizanidine. Implantable intrathecal infusion pumps are another method of controlling spasticity and this can give a sustained improvement in symptoms based on Ashworth scores.

> Spasticity can be seen following stroke and if left untreated can progress to permanent contracture

Botulinum toxin injections are another approach to the management of spasticity. This involves the use of the neuro-toxin derived from botulinum, which is injected into muscle groups to restore a balance between agonist and antagonist muscles across joints. It has been found to be particularly useful when used in elbow flexors, ankle plantar flexors and small limb muscles, such as the intrinsic muscles of the hand.

Epileptic seizures

Seizures occur in approximately 10% of stroke patients and cerebrovascular disease is, therefore, the commonest cause of seizures in the elderly population. Half of these patients develop early seizures (occurring in the first day after stroke) and half are late onset (peak occurring 6–12 months after stroke). Epilepsy

(ie recurrent seizures) occurs in 3–4% of stroke patients. There is a strong correlation between stroke severity and the risk of post-stroke seizure with seizures being more frequent in stroke involving haemorrhage and stroke affecting the cortex. Seizures affecting subcortical structures are still associated with seizure. An agitated confusional state on admission also appears to be an independent risk factor for the development of seizure.

> Cerebrovascular disease is the most common cause of seizures in older people – 10% stroke patients experience a seizure and approximately 4% will have recurrent attacks

The treatment of post-stroke seizures should ideally be a monotherapy as patients will normally have multiple medications with the potential for harmful interactions. The choice of antiepileptic drug would be dependent upon the seizure-type, the characteristics of the patient and other concomitant therapies.

Recurrent stroke

Recurrent stroke is a common complication following the first clinically apparent stroke irrespective of whether it is ischaemic or haemorrhagic. Patients should have risk factors for stroke assessed and any specific secondary prevention measures should be instituted.

Pain after stroke

Pain following stroke may be a result of spasticity, due to dysfunction of the autonomic nervous system, centrally mediated or caused by other specific mechanisms, such as the shoulder–hand syndrome.

Central pain

Centrally generated pain may be associated with thalamic lesions or other central lesions and may present as hemi-body pain with associated allodynia and hyperalgesia. These pains can be very difficult to treat and sometimes require drugs such as the N-methyl-D-aspartate (NMDA) receptor antagonist ketamine. Gabapentin is often used in the first instance and is beneficial in some patients, as is the antidepressant amitriptyline. Carbamazepine and valproate can also be tried.

Complex regional pain syndrome

Complex regional pain syndrome (formerly called sympathetically maintained pain or reflex sympathetic dystrophy) is pain that frequently has a burning-type quality or may be associated with causalgia. This pain sometimes responds to sympathetic nerve block.

> Complex regional pain syndrome following stroke may respond to sympathetic nerve block

Shoulder–hand syndrome

Shoulder–hand syndrome is a common condition that may affect 12.5–27.5% of stroke patients. It is thought to arise after alterations of the biomechanics of the hemiplegic shoulder. The diagnosis is clinical and physical therapies may be the most appropriate means of treating the problem in the initial phase.

Neurogenic heterotopic ossification

Neurogenic heterotopic ossification is an uncommon but important cause of disability and secondary motor disability after neurological injury. Hip, knee and elbow joints seem most commonly affected. The diagnosis is usually established on X-ray and triple-phase bone scan; the erythrocyte sedimentation rate and serum alkaline phosphatase level are also frequently elevated. Non-steroidal anti-inflammatory medications are of some use in a proportion of patients and it is felt that early diagnosis and treatment may be useful (in terms of outcome).

Complications of treatment

Well-established evidence is available to attest to the value of agents used in the secondary prevention of stroke. Every therapy has potential adverse effects. However, strategies can be employed to ensure that the risks of complications of therapy can be minimized.

Antiplatelet agents are used in the secondary prevention of ischaemic stroke. Aspirin, dipyridamole, clopidogrel and ticlopidine have been shown to be effective. The use of aspirin within 48 hours of non-haemorrhagic stroke has been shown to be beneficial, however, the risks of haemorrhagic complications are higher in the acute phase and this needs to be considered when instituting therapy. The risks of gastrointestinal side-effects with aspirin appears to be dose related, yet the efficacy of treatment seems to be as effective using either low- or high-dose regimes. Some doctors advocate the use of proton pump inhibitor prophylaxis if a patient has a history of peptic ulcer disease and is using antiplatelet or anticoagulant therapy. This method attempts to reduce the chances of gastrointestinal haemorrhage occurring.

In those patients intolerant of aspirin, clopidogrel may be an alternative. Evidence from the CAPRIE study showed that clopidogrel may be better tolerated than aspirin in terms of gastrointestinal side-effects, but this was comparing clopidogrel with a relatively high dose of aspirin.

The use of anticoagulants has been shown to be of benefit in specific groups of stroke patients, such as those with atrial fibrillation. Clearly the major risk with anticoagulation is haemorrhage. Maintaining the INR between 2–3 (target INR = 2.5) confers the lowest risk of stroke whilst reducing haemorrhagic complications associated with higher INRs. Reducing the risk of haemorrhagic complications is best achieved by closely monitoring warfarin therapy. This attempts to minimize the time patients might spend outside the therapeutic limits, ie INR <2 or >3. There is evidence of a higher risk of intracranial damage in those patients taking anticoagulants who sustain head injuries; clearly the decision to use anticoagulants in any individual patient must be made on a case-by-case basis, considering the patients risks of falls, their understanding of their medications, etc.

> The major risk when using anticoagulation therapy is haemorrhage. If the INR goes higher than the therapeutic range (ie above 3), the risk of haemorrhage increases

Antihypertensive medications and angiotensin-converting enzyme (ACE) inhibitors in particular are established as a major component in the secondary prevention of stroke. A significant problem with antihypertensive medications is postural hypotension and subsequent falls, especially in the elderly. This problem is important to identify, and unfortunately sometimes requires the withdrawal of medication. Angiotensin-converting enzyme inhibitors in particular may be associated with first-dose postural hypotension and may also precipitate renal failure if there is significant renal artery stenosis. Initiating an ACE-inhibitor at low dose or at night, or by supervising the first dose of an ACE-inhibitor using a short-acting drug (such as captopril) should reduce the associated problems of 'first-dose' hypotension.

Complications following stroke are common and many are preventable. Prevention of complications can improve rates of morbidity and mortality, and hopefully earlier recognition and treatment will result in improved outcome after stroke.

Further reading

Langhorne P. Stott DJ, Robertson L et al. Medical complications after stroke: a multicenter study. *Stroke* 2000; **31**: 1223–9.

Scottish Intercollegiate Guidelines Network. *Management of patients with stroke: rehabilitation, prevention and management of complications, and discharge planning*. SIGN, Edinburgh; Royal College of Physicians of Edinburgh, 2002.

The Intercollegiate Working Party for Stroke. *National Clinical Guidelines for Stroke*. London; Royal College of Physicians, 2000.

10. Rehabilitation after stroke

General principles
What services can the
multidisciplinary team offer?

General principles

Rehabilitation has been defined by the World Health Organization as 'the combined and co-ordinated use of medical, social, educational and vocational measures for training or retraining the individual to the highest level of functional ability'.

Rehabilitation can be an enormous challenge because stroke can be so devastating and have many serious consequences. The benefits of stroke units are well established and one of their most important aspects is their closely integrated rehabilitation team. This multidisciplinary team may be one of the most important factors in the successful outcomes they appear to have. Therapy input must be tailored to the individual patients' needs. The patients with the most severe strokes tend to do less well in terms of outcome when compared to those with mild strokes who make a good spontaneous recovery, even though those with the most severe strokes receive the most input from therapists. Reduction in death and deterioration among patients with moderate to severe strokes is associated with enhanced physiotherapy and occupational therapy input. Speech and language therapy for language problems is required by up to one-third of all surviving stroke patients although most receive less than the optimum amount. Rehabilitation demands a team approach and the different therapy disciplines will approach the patients from different and complementary angles.

The conventional approach to rehabilitation involves a cyclical process of:

- assessment – patients various needs are identified and quantified where possible
- goal setting – goals are defined for improvement (these may be long-/medium-/short-term goals)
- intervention – some form of intervention is provided to try and achieve the goals
- reassessment – progress is assessed against the agreed goals using the same assessment tools where possible.

Rehabilitation goals can be considered at several levels:

- aims – often long-term and may only be achieved after discharge
- objectives – usually multi-professional tackling particular disabilities
- targets – short-term time-limited goals.

The process of rehabilitation can be prejudiced at any stage by previous disability, comorbidities and complications of the stroke itself.

Assessment of the individual's rehabilitation needs is essential. This involves the collection of data about the disability and their interpretation. Disability can be measured using standardized scales. Scales measuring neurological impairment include the NIH stroke scale, Orgogozo neurological score and more modern developments. Scales measuring activities of daily living include the Barthel index; more complex activities can be measured by instrumental (or extended) activities of daily living scales. These domains have been combined in scales such as the Functional Independence Measure. Handicap can be measured by the Rankin scale, more often expressed as the modified Rankin scale or Oxford Handicap scale. Mental function can be measured with an Abbreviated Mental Test Score, Mental Status Questionnaire or Mini Mental Test Score. Clearly a pragmatic approach using a selection of these instruments should be used in clinical practice.

> Every stroke patient should be assessed for neurological function (NIH stroke scale), disability (Barthel index), handicap (modified Rankin score) and mental status

A team approach is essential in rehabilitation and the aims have to be realistic. Goal setting is one of the specific characteristics of rehabilitation. It refers to a common target which the team will work toward over a specified period of time. Goals need to be reset depending on outcomes and need to be both short-term and long-term. In practice different approaches to individual patients' specific needs will be required. No one single approach has been found to be more effective than others.

The multidisciplinary team responsible for stroke patients should consist of appropriate levels of nursing, medical, physiotherapy, occupational therapy, speech and language therapy, and social work staff. Other disciplines are regularly involved in the management of stroke patients including clinical psychologists, psychiatrists and dieticians.

Important principles in rehabilitation include:

- Early mobilization – which is promoted to prevent a number of complications associated with immobility.
- Intensity of therapy input. The optimum amount of therapy input is not known. Trials have not adequately addressed this question.

What services can the multidisciplinary team offer?

Nursing care

Stroke nursing is a specialist branch of nursing. Stroke nurses have the knowledge, skills and interest to deliver effective therapeutic care and rehabilitation (this requires education and training in stroke care). Stroke nurses focus on working in partnership with the patient and his/her family, involving them in decision making and taking responsibility for their own recovery. Stroke nurses take into account the holistic needs of the patient and family, involving the physical, psychological and social aspects of care. As each patient and family is unique, stroke nurses consider the individual's needs. Stroke nursing is a continuous 24-hour process throughout the patient's journey, wherever the setting – whether in an acute unit, a rehabilitation unit or at home. The organization of nursing practice, eg primary nursing, is an enabling factor to effective stroke care as part of a multidisciplinary team.

> The multidisciplinary team consists of stroke nurses, physicians, GPs, dieticians, speech & language therapists, physiotherapists, occupational therapists, social workers, psychologists and surgeons

Physician

The physician members of the stroke multidisciplinary team will comprise consultant(s) and other career-grade physicians and trainees at various stages of training. Roles will vary depending on experience and responsibility. The physician should have a background and training in general medicine, clinical pharmacology, geriatric medicine, neurology or rehabilitation medicine, and would be able to call on the skills of colleagues when referral is appropriate.

The general role of the physician (as defined by the British Association of Stroke Physicians) is to lead, coordinate and develop the skills and decisions of the multidisciplinary team. Physicians will understand the concept of multidisciplinary working in stroke rehabilitation and the criteria for successful multidisciplinary working. There will be an appreciation of the roles of other professionals within stroke rehabilitation and an in-depth understanding of the role of the stroke physician within multidisciplinary stroke rehabilitation. Particular skills and responsibilities will be appropriate to the nature and emphasis of the stroke unit (eg acute or rehabilitation).

General practitioner

The GP also has an integral role in the multi-disciplinary management of patients with stroke. GPs working in a community setting have particular strengths in problem solving, treating co-morbidities in the patient and helping carers who may have illnesses of their own to cope with in addition to caring. GPs have a role in coordinating the various services, including hospital-based services, social services and professions allied to medicine. The GP is responsible for key decisions at certain points in the patient journey such as whether to and where to admit the patient. The GP is solely responsible for and accountable for prescribing to patients in the community. The GP role is critical at the time of first diagnosis when the decisions regarding further investigation and possible admission have to be made with the patient and the carers. Their experience in the availability of local resources will be invaluable.

> GPs have an important role in treating co-morbidities and aiding carers who may also have illnesses of their own to deal with

When admission is being contemplated, the GP should tell the hospital staff the basis of the diagnosis, the premorbid condition of the patient, any relevant social factors and past medical history. The GP's role is also pivotal in the discharge of patients back to the community. These patients often have a complex treatment and rehabilitation strategy with multiple co-morbidities. The GP will be responsible for continuing secondary prevention.

Physiotherapy

Physiotherapists are experts in the assessment and treatment of movement disorders. Physiotherapy involves the skilled use of physical interventions (as opposed to medicine or surgery) in order to restore functional movement or reduce impairment, disability and handicap after injury or disease. These physical interventions commonly involve exercise and movement and may include the use of thermal or electrical treatments. Physiotherapists are generally involved in the care and rehabilitation of patients from the time of onset of the stroke. Their input may often be daily and may last for many months and, in some cases, years. The input can take place in a variety of settings including stroke units, acute admission wards, general medical wards, rehabilitation units, day hospitals, community day centres, out-patient clinics and the patient's own home.

An important part of physiotherapy is full assessment at the earliest opportunity, and to carry out on-going assessments throughout the rehabilitation process. Use of recognized assessment scales facilitates this; key elements include:

- respiratory function
- muscle tone
- body alignment and range of joint motion
- movement status
- sensation
- visuospatial awareness
- undesirable compensatory activity
- balance
- mobility – walking, transfers, stair-climbing.

> Physiotherapy begins after stroke and promotes early mobilization in the rehabilitation process

Physiotherapy aims to restore normal functional movement by promoting early mobilization and the use of motor learning programmes. The techniques used tend to be goal orientated and task specific. Treatment aims to recruit spared neural pathways, and full concentration and repetition of exercises are required from the patient if they are to improve.

Physiotherapy aims to prevent soft-tissue shortening and adaptive changes. Physiotherapists are expert in minimizing and managing spasticity by:

- mobilization of soft tissue
- promoting correct symmetry
- promoting good handling
- splinting
- positioning
- use of drugs.

There is no available evidence to suggest that any one specific physiotherapy technique is superior to any other in terms of outcome. Good communication between the physiotherapist and other members of the multidisciplinary team is important. More physiotherapy input is associated with a reduction in deterioration and death.

Occupational therapy

Occupational therapists assess and treat people who have impairments, restricted activity levels and limited ability to participate as a result of injury or illness, in order to achieve the highest level of independence possible.

The occupational therapist will identify the individual aspects that make up a person's ability to carry out selected activities (ie physical, cognitive, perceptual, psychological, social and environmental aspects) and will include jointly agreed goals and purposeful activity in their interventions. Purposeful activity is used to minimize disability and to promote the restoration and maximum use of function to help individuals return to their usual levels of activity in the domains of self-maintenance, productivity and leisure activity. Occupational therapy should also begin from the time of onset of the stroke (or as soon as is

practical). Intervention can last from months to years with rehabilitation commencing in an acute stroke unit and following patients through into the community setting and at home.

> Occupational therapy should begin as soon as is practical after stroke onset and aims to restore the highest level of independence that is possible

The key elements of occupational therapy with stroke patients include:

- assessment of skills for the performance of self care (eg washing, dressing, feeding), domestic ability (eg shopping, cooking, cleaning), work and leisure occupations
- assessment of skills which impact on present activity (eg sensori-motor, cognitive, perceptual and psychosocial impairments)
- using activity analysis, in which the components of an activity are identified along with the individual's limitations in carrying it out
- assessment of social environment (eg family, friends, relationships)
- assessment of physical environment (eg home and workplace).

Interventions are complementary to those of other therapists and are aimed to:

- help each patient achieve the highest level of independence possible and to minimize disability
- regain physical, sensory, cognitive and perceptual skills through activity and practice
- promote the use of purposeful, goal-orientated activities to improve quality of life and sense of wellbeing
- teach new strategies and compensatory techniques to aid independence (eg memory aids, splints, orthotic and prosthetic devices and wheelchairs)
- assess, advise and install appropriate equipment and adaptations to enhance

independent function (eg bath aids, wheelchairs)

- assess for and provide appropriate seating and to advise on positioning
- assess, advise and facilitate transport and mobility issues such as driving
- facilitate the transfer of care from acute stages (eg in hospital) through rehabilitation (in hospital or community) and discharge (to home or continuing-care facility)
- liaise, work with and refer to other professionals as part of a multidisciplinary team
- educate the patient and carer in all relevant aspects of stroke care
- liaise with support groups and voluntary bodies.

Speech and language therapy

The role of the speech and language therapist in the rehabilitation of stroke is wide-ranging. It will include the provision of a diagnostic service for both swallowing and communication – assessing, in the acute phase, swallowing and its problems (oral and pharyngeal) and communication impairment (dysphasia, dysarthria and dyspraxia). Provision of information to patients, carers and healthcare staff about impairments/disabilities, related abilities, recommended feeding regimes and the facilitation of communication is another responsibility of the speech and language therapist. An appropriate speech and language therapy care programme will be set up, which may include support, regular therapy and possibly intensive therapy. This programme facilitates access to information regarding methods of coping with swallowing and speech problems, therapies available, exploring new methods of communication (including augmentative and alternative communication systems) and accessing support groups, see Appendix I.

One-third of all surviving stroke patients will require the services of a speech and language therapist, but the majority of these patients

will receive less than 45 minutes per week of such therapy.

> Speech and language therapy is required by one-third of stroke survivors, but most of these patients spend less than 45 minutes with a therapist each week

Social worker

The social worker is employed by the local authority and has an understanding of the illness and its effect on the patient, carers and family. As well as being aware of the physical problems of a stroke, the social worker will also be aware of the psychological and emotional impacts of stroke illness so that he/she can best understand the patient's needs.

The social worker works closely with individual members of the multidisciplinary team and is especially aware of therapists' reports when determining the needs of the patient. Social workers become involved with patients at different stages of the rehabilitation process, depending on what problems the patient and their family may have. Advice and information may be required at an early stage and the social worker has useful skills in helping with financial, relationship or housing problems.

The social worker needs to have a wide knowledge of resources in the community so that he/she is able to advise the team and the patient about what is available for the patient on discharge. It is the social worker's role to advise the team about the timescale for implementing care packages and to discuss alternative forms of care if required.

> Social workers have good knowledge of the resources available to stroke patients within a community. They can advise the rest of the multidisciplinary team, thereby helping them to decide how to treat each patient after discharge

As the time for discharge approaches, the social worker will normally become more involved with patients and especially those who have complex needs. The social worker will complete community care assessments for patients and will consult with the multidisciplinary team, the patient and their family. It is important for the social worker to be aware of the patient's own goals and expectations and to be able to assess any risk that the patient may be in. The social worker will then organize the appropriate care, either in the community or in residential homes as may be required. The social worker will then go on to work with the patient and family for a period of time after discharge to ensure that rehabilitation plans are meeting their needs and to support patients and families in organizing and re-assessing any difficult situations that may arise.

Clinical psychologist

In the UK the majority of stroke patients do not have the opportunity to benefit from the input of a clinical psychologist. They are expert in dealing with emotional and personality changes. They can help by providing neuropsychological assessment and treatment strategies for:

- intellectual and cognitive impairment
- behavioural problems
- daily functioning
- interpersonal and emotional problems.

Vascular surgeon

Close liaison with a vascular surgeon is required when carotid endarterectomy is contemplated. Their expertise and advice in preparation for any surgery that is being considered is appreciated.

Dietician

The dietician has a role in maintaining adequate nutrition for the stroke patient.

Swallowing problems may mean that specially thickened feeds are required. In addition, feeding regimes for nasogastric feeding and percutaneous gastrostomy tube feeding will be tailored by the dietician. Malnutrition in stroke patients is associated with a poor outcome.

> Dieticians are a useful part of the multidisciplinary team as swallowing problems and insertion of feeding tubes are common after stroke, and malnutrition is linked to a poor outcome

Other members of the multidisciplinary team

Depending on individual patient circumstances other members might include a psychiatrist, a chiropodist, a dentist, a chaplain and an optician. Often the clinicians responsible for the stroke patient's care will consult with other specialists for advice. Patients and carers should be involved at an early stage as active members of the multidisciplinary team.

Further reading

Ernst E. A review of stroke rehabilitation and physiotherapy. *Stroke* 1990; **21**: 1081–5.

Fialka Moser V, Ward AB. Commentary on the scope for rehabilitation in severely disabled stroke patients. *Disabil Rehabil* 2000; **22**: 188–92; discussion 205.

Hill S, Main A. Therapeutic progress – review XXIII. Are we making progress in the treatment of acute stroke? *J Clin Hosp Pharm* 1986; **11**: 427–41.

Hochstenbach J, Mulder T. Neuropsychology and the relearning of motor skills following stroke. *Int J Rehabil Res* 1999; **22**: 11–19.

Langhorne P, Dennis M (Eds). *Stroke Units: An Evidence Based Approach*. BMJ Books: London, 1998.

Sellars C, Hughes T, Langhorne P. Speech and language therapy for dysarthria due to nonprogressive brain damage: a systematic Cochrane review. *Clin Rehabil* 2002; **16**: 61–8.

Sulch D, Kalra L. Integrated care pathways in stroke management. *Age Ageing* 2000; **29**: 349–52.

Warner R. The effectiveness of nursing in stroke units. *Nursing Standard* 2000; **14**: 32–5.

11. Stroke services

Hospital- or home-based care?
Organization of hospital care
Discharge
Community rehabilitation
Local stroke services – planning and
delivery

Until recently, services for stroke survivors have been haphazard, and poorly organized and coordinated. Over the past 12 years there has been increasing evidence of service strategies proven to benefit stroke patients in terms of optimizing survival and outcome.

Trials of services for stroke patients have focussed on broad policy decisions (eg whether to admit patients to hospital or manage them at home), and have compared sometimes ill-defined and diverse services with each other. Trials have often been in carefully selected patient groups and so their outcomes are not applicable to most stroke patients.

When a patient suffers a stroke, a series of clinical decisions will follow (either implicit or explicit) regarding the most appropriate setting for their care. These decisions will be influenced by local variables and potential solutions. Efficient and effective management of patients depends on a well-organized expert service that can respond to the particular needs of each individual patient. The organization of a stroke service must therefore be considered at the level of the health authority or board, Primary Care Trust (PCT), hospital ward and in the patient's own home.

> Organization of the application of stroke services covers the local health authority, PCT, hospital ward and the patient's home

The four key points in managing a stroke patient are as follows:

- hospital- or home-based care?
- organization of hospital care
- discharge and post-discharge services
- ongoing rehabilitation and follow-up.

Hospital- or home-based care?

While patients with mild stroke and transient ischaemic attacks (TIAs) can often be managed as outpatients (if adequate facilities are available), patients with more severe symptoms are more appropriately referred to hospital for acute assessment and rehabilitation.

> Patients who suffer a stroke should be treated as an emergency. This means assessment and management in hospital in all but the mildest cases. Mobile patients should be referred to an adequately resourced outpatient facility

Non-disabling stroke

Patients who have a non-disabling stroke need to be urgently investigated and this may be most efficiently done by either immediate admission to hospital or by early access to a neurovascular clinic. To avoid missing small primary intracerebral haemorrhage and the rare but devastating causes of stroke (such as bacterial endocarditis), computerized tomography scanning should be performed within 48 hours.

More severe strokes

Trials in mild to moderate stroke patients comparing management at home, including input from multidisciplinary domiciliary care teams (offering the level of care provided in hospital), with hospital care have failed to show a benefit for home-based care. Treatment at home has not shown any reduction in hospital bed use, due to the number of 'rescue' admissions to hospital. A later trial by Kalra and colleagues compared domiciliary care to two types of hospital care (general wards with a stroke team giving advice and an organized stroke unit). Stroke outcome was significantly better when patients were treated in the organized hospital stroke unit compared with organized domiciliary care or general ward hospital care (with stroke team advice). Treatment at home as an alternative to initial assessment admission is not justified.

Stroke patients who need help to mobilize or who are dependent in activities of daily living (ADL) should receive hospital-based organized stroke unit care.

Organization of hospital care

It has been shown in several settings that acute treatment of stroke, especially in stroke units, definitely improves outcome and lowers mortality after stroke. In two trials comparing care at home with care in a stroke unit there was clear superiority for the stroke units. In the 23 randomized trials comparing stroke units with general wards there was superiority of outcome (including reduction in mortality and need for institutional care) from the stroke units.

> Acute treatment in hospital stroke units improves outcome and reduces mortality after stroke

The characteristics of the individual stroke units differed in the trials. The stroke unit care philosophy includes core processes and procedures based around a coordinated multidisciplinary team of personnel who are specifically trained in stroke care. The specialist staff undergo a continuous programme of education and training enabling them to facilitate coordinated multidisciplinary care (for prolonged periods if necessary). Stroke units of

all types have advantages over 'normal' inpatient wards – the configuration may be acute, comprehensive (acute and rehabilitation), rehabilitation only, including rehabilitation in a purely stroke ward or a mixed rehabilitation ward. The comprehensive stroke units, commonly seen in Scandinavia, have the best evidence base for their superiority over general wards. A mobile stroke team, although offering some of the advantages of a stroke unit, has been proven to be of limited benefit compared to a properly configured and operated stroke unit. Organized stroke care (provided by a multidisciplinary team based in a stroke unit) results in more patients surviving, returning home and regaining independence. It is not clear which particular 'ingredients' of the stroke unit 'recipe' are the most important to the improved outcomes.

Among the benefits of stroke rehabilitation in an organized hospital stroke unit are:

- a reduction in death (18% odds reduction; 95% confidence interval [CI] 6–29)
- a reduction in death or institutional care (20% odds reduction; 95% CI 10–29)
- a reduction in death or dependency (22% odds reduction; 95% CI 11–32).

These benefits were seen for those under and over 75 years of age, male and female, and for those with mild, moderate or severe stroke. Length of stay appears to have been reduced by between two and 10 days but this result is inconsistent between trials. There was certainly no systematic increase in length of hospital stay.

> The benefits of stroke rehabilitation in an organized stroke unit are seen in all age groups, in both sexes and in mild, moderate and severe stroke patients

The benefits of a stroke unit were seen for those units that admitted patients directly from the community or took over their care within two weeks of admission to hospital. The numbers needed to treat for stroke unit care can be stated as:

- For every 33 (95% CI 20–100) patients treated in the stroke unit, there is one extra survivor.
- For every 20 (95% CI 12–50) patients treated in the stroke unit, one extra patient is discharged back to their own home.
- For every 20 (95% CI 12–50) patients treated in the stroke unit, there is one extra independent survivor.

The confidence intervals are wide and suggest benefits may vary from modest to substantial depending on the success of individual stroke units. These data suggest that further improvements in the quality of care are feasible.

Rehabilitation needs of younger adults with stroke may include vocational rehabilitation and caring for a young family. There is some evidence that input from specialists in rehabilitation of younger adults is helpful. When stroke unit care is not possible then rehabilitation in an effective rehabilitation ward may be the best alternative choice.

> Young adults who suffer a stroke need input from specialists who deal with rehabilitation needs of young people – they advise on, eg caring for a young family and vocational rehabilitation

Discharge

Carefully planned discharge after an admission for acute stroke is sensible to facilitate good management in the community. However, studies of planned discharge have shown mixed results. These studies have not been restricted to stroke populations and have been implemented in different ways. There is some evidence that discharge planning may lead to reduced length of stay in hospital, and in some cases reduced readmission rate to hospital.

There is also some evidence that discharge planning increases patient satisfaction.

Community rehabilitation
Early supported discharge

Community rehabilitation teams catering for patients at home as an alternative to early admission have not been as successful as early admission and hospital assessment in meeting patients' needs. However, there is growing evidence that (after appropriate stroke unit care) early supported discharge for selected patients is possible and may be superior to conventional discharge. Services aiming to accelerate discharge and provide rehabilitation within the home setting must be well coordinated and delivered. Trials from the UK, Norway, Sweden, Australia, Canada and the USA suggest that hospital length of stay can be reduced by an average of nine days (95% CI 5–15; p<0.0001). However, early supported discharge schemes are not applicable to all stroke patients – they are usually only useful for those with a degree of independence and/or a supportive relative at home, and most services excluded those with very mild or very severe stroke. The schemes in the studies were available for approximately 30% of all hospitalized stroke patients. This means that only carefully selected patients currently appear to benefit.

> Only 30% of stroke patients would be eligible for an early supported discharge scheme

Early supported discharge services provided by a well-resourced, coordinated multidisciplinary team are an acceptable alternative to more prolonged hospital stroke unit care. These services can reduce the length of hospital stay for selected patients

Follow-up
Further rehabilitation at home

There is some evidence that there may be small improvements in ADL scores and reductions in deterioration when further rehabilitation input is given at home after discharge. Physiotherapy at one year after a stroke can result in small improvements which are not sustained when therapy is withdrawn.

Stroke liaison worker

After discharge, input from stroke liaison workers may improve the emotional outcome of carers. These people may or may not have a nursing background.

Local stroke services – planning and delivery

Stroke services have to be carefully tailored to meet local needs. This applies to those patients who have to be admitted for assessment and those who can be evaluated at a rapid-access cerebrovascular clinic. Figure 11.1 shows an example of a local stroke-care

pathway. Once the decision to admit the patient is made, local circumstances will dictate where the patient is managed. A properly staffed and resourced stroke unit with a multidisciplinary team will achieve the best outcomes. Proper services should be available on discharge to aid the transition back in to the community.

Figure 11.2 shows where stroke patients should be managed. For patients with a severe or moderately severe stroke, the usual option is to admit them to hospital; for those with milder strokes, early hospitalization for multidisciplinary assessment and treatment may be valuable. For mild-stroke patients who are mobile and for patients with a TIA, there should be fast-track assessment clinics available to allow these patients to be managed effectively by the appropriate experts. A considerable investment will be required throughout the UK to achieve this.

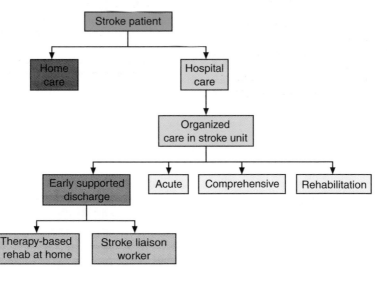

Figure 11.1
Local services model for acute stroke patients.

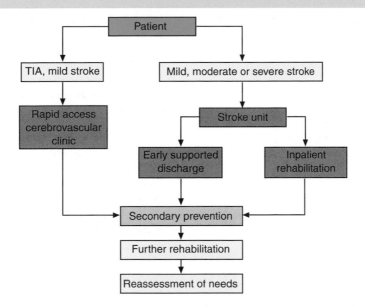

Figure 11.2
Model for management of TIA and stroke patients of various severities.

TIA, transient ischaemic attack

Further reading

Anderson CS, Linto J, Stewart-Wynne EG. A population-based assessment of the impact and burden of caregiving for long-term stroke survivors. *Stroke* 1995; **26**: 843–9.

Dewey HM, Thrift AG, Mihalopoulos C *et al*. Cost of stroke in Australia from a societal perspective: results from the North East Melbourne Stroke Incidence Study (NEMESIS). *Stroke* 2001; **32**: 2409–16.

Langhorne P. Organisation of acute stroke care. *Br Med Bull* 2000; **56**: 436–43.

Mant J, Carter J, Wade DT, Winner S. Family support for stroke: a randomised controlled trial. *Lancet* 2000; **356**: 808–13.

Neau JP, Paquereau J, Meurice JC *et al*. Stroke and sleep apnoea: cause or consequence? *Sleep Med Rev* 2002; **6**: 457–69.

Rodgers H, Soutter J, Kaiser W *et al*. Early supported hospital discharge following acute stroke: pilot study results. *Clin Rehabil* 1997; **11**: 280–7.

Shepperd S, Iliffe S. Hospital at home versus in-patient hospital care. *Cochrane Database Syst Rev* 2001; **3**: CD000356.

Tyson S, Turner G. Discharge and follow up for people with stroke: what happens and why. *Clin Rehabil* 2000; **14**: 381–92.

Appendix I: Useful addresses

The following organizations provide support and information for stroke patients and their carers:

British Association for Counselling and Psychotherapy
1 Regent Place
Rugby
Warwickshire CV21 2PJ
Tel: 0870 443 5252
Fax: 0870 443 5160
Web: www.counselling.co.uk

Carers National Association Scotland
91 Mitchell Street
Glasgow G1 3LN
Tel: 0141 221 9141
Fax: 0141 221 9140
Carers Line: 0345 573 369
Email: internet@carerscotland.demon.co.uk

Chest, Heart & Stroke Scotland
65 North Castle Street
Edinburgh EH2 3LT
Advice Line: 0845 077 6000
Tel: 0131 225 6963
Fax: 0131 220 6313
Email: admin@chss.org.uk
Web: www.chss.org.uk

Connect (Communication Disability Network)
16–18 Marshalsea Road
London SE1 1HL
Tel: 020 7367 0840
Fax: 020 7347 0841
Email: info@ukconnect.org
Web: www.ukconnect.org

Different Strokes
Sir Walter Scott House
PO Box 5082
Milton Keynes MK5 7HZ
Tel: 01908 236 033
Fax: 01908 236 032
Email: info@differentstrokes.co.uk
Web: www.differentstrokes.co.uk

Disabled Living Foundation
380–384 Harrow Road
London W9 2HU
Tel: 020 7286 6111
Web: www.dlf.org.uk

KEYCOMM
Lothian Communication Technology Service
St Giles Centre
40 Broomhouse Crescent
Edinburgh EH11 3UB
Tel: 0131 443 6775
Fax: 0131 443 5121
Email: djans@keycomm.demon.co.uk

Moving Intowork
(Employment consultancy and support for people after acquired brain injury)
Norton Park
57 Albion Road
Edinburgh EH7 5QY;
Braid House
Labrador Avenue
Howden
Livingston EH54 6AU
Email: moving@intowork.org.uk
Web: www.intowork.org.uk/moving

Northern Ireland Chest, Heart & Stroke Association
21 Dublin Road
Belfast BT2 7HB
Tel: 028 9032 0184
Fax: 028 9033 3487
Web: www.nichsa.com

Princess Royal Trust for Carers
(Glasgow Office)
Campbell House
215 West Campbell Street
Glasgow G2 4TT
Tel: 0141 221 5066
Fax: 0141 221 4623
Email: infoscotland@carers.org
Web: www.carers.org

Rehab Scotland
Head Office
1650 London Road
Glasgow G31 4QF.
Tel: 0141 554 8822
Email: headoffice@rehab-scotland.co.uk
Web: www.rehab.ie/scotland/index.htm

**Royal Association for Disability and
Rehabilitation (RADAR)**
12 City Forum
250 City Road
London EC1V 8AF
Tel: 020 7250 3222
Fax: 020 7250 0212
Email: radar@radar.org.uk
Web: www.radar.org.uk

**Scottish Centre of Technology for the
Communication Impaired**
SCTCI
WESTMARC
Southern General Hospital
1345 Govan Road
Glasgow G51 4TF
Tel: 0141 201 2619
Fax: 0141 201 2618
Email: sctci@waacis.edex.co.uk

**Shaw Trust (helps people with disabilities
return to work)**
Shaw House
Epsom Square
White Horse Business Park
Trowbridge BA14 0XJ
Tel: 01225 716350
Fax: 01225 716334
Email: stir@shaw-trust.org.uk
Web: www.shaw-trust.org.uk

Society for Research in Rehabilitation
Division of Stroke Medicine
Clinical Science Building
Nottingham City Hospital
Hucknall Road
Nottingham NG5 1PB
Tel: 0115 840 4798
Fax: 0115 840 4790
Web: www.srr.org.uk

Speakability (information for people with
aphasia, their families and healthcare
professionals)
1 Royal Street
London SE1 7LL
Helpline: 080 8808 9572
Tel: 020 7261 9522
Fax: 020 7928 9542
Web: www.speakability.org.uk

The Stroke Association
Stroke House
Whitecross Street
London EC1Y 8JJ
Tel: 020 7566 0300
Fax 020 7490 2686
Web: www.stroke.org.uk

Appendix II: Stroke scales

National Institutes of Health stroke scale
Unified neurological stroke scale
Barthel index
Modified Rankin scale
Instrumental activities of daily living
Geriatric depression scale
MRC clinical grading scale

National Institutes of Health stroke scale

The National Institutes of Health stroke scale is used to assess the degree of neurological deficit after an acute stroke. Important points on the National Institutes of Health (NIH) stroke scale include:

- Each examination is assessed independently from previous examinations.
- A response must be checked for each item, using the following definitions:
  - 1a Level of consciousness
  - 1b Level of consciousness – questions
  - 1c Level of consciousness – commands
  - 2 Gaze
  - 3 Visual field
  - 4 Facial movement (facial paresis)
  - 5 Motor function – arms (left and right arm)
  - 6 Motor function – legs (left and right leg)
  - 7 Limb ataxia
  - 8 Sensory
  - 9 Best language
  - 10 Dysarthria
  - 11 Neglect (extinction and inattention).

NIH stroke scale	
1a Level of consciousness	0 Alert
	1 Not alert, but arousable with minimal stimulation
	2 Not alert, requires repeated stimulation to attend
	3 Coma
1b Ask patient the month and their age	0 Answers both correctly
	1 Answers one correctly
	2 Both incorrect
1c Ask patient to open and close eyes	0 Obeys both correctly
	1 Obeys one correctly
	2 Both incorrect
2 Best gaze (only horizontal eye movement)	0 Normal
	1 Partial gaze palsy
	2 Forced deviation
3 Visual field testing	0 No visual field loss
	1 Partial hemianopia
	2 Complete hemianopia
	3 Bilateral hemianopia (blind including cortical blindness)

continued

continued

4 Facial paresis (ask patient to show teeth or raise eyebrows and close eyes tightly)	0 Normal symmetrical movement 1 Minor paralysis (flattened nasolabial fold, asymmetry on smiling) 2 Partial paralysis (total or near total paralysis of lower face) 3 Complete paralysis of one or both sides (absence of facial movement in the upper and lower face)
5 Motor function – arm (right and left) Right arm _____ Left arm _____	0 Normal (extends arms 90° [or 45°] for 10 seconds without drift) 1 Drift 2 Some effort against gravity 3 No effort against gravity 4 No movement 9 Untestable (joint fused or limb amputated)
6 Motor function – leg (right and left) Right leg _____ Left leg _____	0 Normal (hold leg in 30° position for 5 seconds) 1 Drift 2 Some effort against gravity 3 No effort against gravity 4 No movement 9 Untestable (joint fused or limb amputated)
7 Limb ataxia	0 No ataxia 1 Present in one limb 2 Present in two limbs
8 Sensory (use pinprick to test arms, legs, trunk and face – compare side to side)	0 Normal 1 Mild to moderate decrease in sensation 2 Severe to total sensory loss
9 Best language (describe picture, name items, read sentences)	0 No aphasia 1 Mild to moderate aphasia 2 Severe aphasia 3 Mute
10 Dysarthria (read several words)	0 Normal articulation 1 Mild to moderate slurring of words 2 Near unintelligible or unable to speak 9 Intubated or other physical barrier
11 Neglect (extinction and inattention)	0 Normal 1 Inattention or extinction to bilateral simultaneous stimulation in one of the sensory modalities 2 Severe hemi-inattention or hemi-inattention to more than one modality

General instructions for use of NIH stroke scale

1a Level of consciousness

This global measure of responsiveness is assessed by the patient's interactions with the physician at the bedside when the patient is first examined. The physician should stimulate the patient (by patting or tapping the patient) to determine the best level of consciousness. On occasion, more noxious stimuli, such as pinching, may be required to check the level of consciousness.

0 = Alert – patient is fully alert and keenly responsive.

1 = Drowsy – patient is drowsy but can be aroused with minor stimulation. The patient

obeys, answers and responds to commands.

2 = Stuporous – patient is lethargic but requires repeated stimulation to attend. The patient may need painful or strong stimuli to respond to or follow commands.

3 = Coma – patient is comatose and responds only with reflexive motor or automatic responses. Otherwise, the patient is unresponsive.

1b Level of conciousness – questions

Level of consciousness – questions is checked by asking the patient to respond to two questions. The patient is asked the month of the year and his/her age. The answer must be correct – there is no partial credit for being close (for example, being out by one year in age). If the patient gives the wrong initial answer but then corrects it, the answer should still be scored as incorrect. Other measures of orientation such as time of day, location, etc. are not asked as part of this examination. If the patient has aphasia, the physician should judge the responses to questions in light of the language impairment.

0 = answers BOTH correctly.

1 = Answers ONE correctly.

2 = BOTH incorrect.

1c Level of conciousness – commands

The level of consciousness – commands is checked by asking the patient to follow two commands. The patient is asked to open and close their eyes and then is asked to make a grip (close and open their hand). Only the initial response is scored. If a patient is aphasic and unable to follow verbal commands, the patient may imitate these movements (pantomime). For a patient who has hemiparesis, the response in the unaffected limb should be measured. For example, if the patient has a left hemiparesis, making a fist with the right hand is a normal response to the command. If a paralysed patient does try to move the limb in response to a command but is unable to form a fist, it is counted as a normal response.

0 = Obeys BOTH correctly.

1 = Obeys ONE correctly.

2 = BOTH incorrect.

2 Gaze

The position of the eyes at rest and movement of the eyes to command are tested. First look at the position of the eyes at rest. Spontaneous eye movements to the left or right should be noted. The patient is then asked to look to the left or right. Only horizontal eye movements are tested. Disorders of vertical gaze, nystagmus or skew deviation are not measured. Reflexive eye movements (oculocephalic or oculovestibular) should be tested in patients who are unable to respond to commands. If a patient has ocular rotatory problems, such as a strabismus, but leaves the midline and attempts to look both right and left, he/she should be considered to have a normal response. If a patient has an isolated oculorotatory problem, such as an oculomotor (CN III) or abducens (CN IV) palsy, the score should be 1. If the patient has a conjugate deviation of the eyes that can be overcome by voluntary or reflexive activity, the score should be 1. If there is a conjugate lateral deviation that is NOT overcome with reflexive movements, the score should be 2.

0 = Normal – the patient has normal lateral eye movements.

1 = Partial gaze palsy – patient is unable to move one or both eyes completely to both directions.

2 = Forced deviation – patient has conjugate deviation of the eyes to the right or left, even with reflexive movements.

3 Visual fields

Visual fields of both eyes are examined. In most cases, the physician asks the patient to count fingers in all four quadrants. Each eye is independently tested. If a patient is unable to respond verbally, the physician should check responses (attending) to visual stimuli in the quadrants or have the patient hold up the number of fingers seen. A quadrantic field cut should be scored 1. The entire half field (both upper and lower quadrants) should be involved with a dense field loss and is scored 2. If a patient has severe monocular visual loss due to intrinsic eye disease and the visual fields in the other eye as normal, the physician should score the visual fields as normal. If the patient has monocular blindness due to primary eye disease and the visual fields in the other 'normal' eye demonstrate a partial or dense visual field defect, the visual loss should be scored as 1, 2 or 3 as appropriate.

0 = No visual loss.

1 = Partial hemianopia – there is a partial visual field defect in both eyes. Included is a quadrantic field defect or sector field defect.

2 = Complete hemianopia – there is dense visual field defect in both eyes. A homonymous hemianopia is included.

3 = Bilateral hemianopia – there are bilateral visual field defects in both eyes. Cortical blindness is included.

4 Facial movement (facial paresis)

This is examined by looking at the patient's face and noting any spontaneous facial movements. The facial movements in response to commands are also tested. Such commands may include asking the patient to grimace or smile, to puff out his/her cheeks, to pucker and to close his/her eyes forcefully. If the patient is aphasic and is unable to follow commands, the physician should have the patient attempt imitative (pantomime) responses. The facial responses to painful stimuli (grimace) may substitute for responses to commands in a patient who has decreased levels of alertness.

0 = Normal facial movements – no asymmetry.

1 = Minor paresis – asymmetrical facial movements or facial asymmetry at rest. This response may be noted with a spontaneous smile but not with forced facial movements.

2 = Partial paresis – unilateral 'central' facial paresis. Decreased spontaneous and forced

facial movements with changes most prominent at the mouth. Orbital and forehead musculature movements are normal.

3 = Complete palsy – dysfunction involves forehead, orbital and circumoral muscles (the entire distribution of the facial nerve). Deficits may be unilateral or bilateral (facial diplegia) complete facial paresis.

5 Motor function – arms (right and left)

The patient is asked to extend their arm in front of the body at 90° (if sitting) or at 45° (if supine). The effort is for a full 10 seconds. The physician should count to ten aloud to encourage the patient to maintain the limb's position. If a limb is paralysed, the physician may wish to test any 'normal' limb first. If a patient is aphasic, directions may be achieved by non-verbal cues or pantomime. Patients may be 'helped' by the physician by placing the limb in the desired position. If the patient has restricted limb function due to arthritis or non-stroke related limitations, the physician should attempt to judge the 'best' motor response. If the patient has decreased level of consciousness, an estimate of response to noxious stimuli should be measured. Volitional motor responses that are performed well should be graded as 0. If the patient has reflexive responses, such as flexor or extensor posturing, the response should be scored as 4. The only indications for scoring this item as 9 (untestable) are when the limb is missing or amputated, or if the shoulder joint is fused. A patient with a partial limb amputation should be tested.

0 = No drift – the patient is able to hold the outstretched limb for 10 seconds.

1 = Drift – the patient is able to hold the outstretched limb for 10 seconds but there is some fluttering or drift of the limb. If the limb falls to an intermediate position, the score is 1.

2 = Some effort against gravity – the patient is not able to hold the outstretched limb for 10 seconds but there is some effort against gravity.

3 = No effort against gravity – the patient is not able to bring the limb off the bed but there is some effort against gravity. If the limb is raised in the correct position by the examiner, the patient is unable to sustain the position.

4 = No movement – the patient is unable to move the limb. There is no effort against gravity.

9 = Untestable – may only be used if the limb is missing or amputated, or if the shoulder joint is fused.

6 Motor function – leg (right and left)

The supine patient is asked to hold the outstretched leg at 30° above the bed. The limb should be held in this position for five seconds. The physician should count to five aloud to encourage the patient to maintain the limb's position. If the right leg is paralysed, the examiner may wish to examine the 'normal' left leg first. If a patient is unable to follow verbal commands nonverbal cues may be used or the limb may be placed in the desired position. If the patient has a decreased level of consciousness, an estimate of response to noxious stimuli should be measured. Volitional motor responses that are performed well should be scored 0. If the patient has reflexive responses, such as flexor or extensor posturing, the response should be scored 4. The only indication for scoring this item as 9 (untestable) is if the limb is missing or if the hip joint is fused. Patients with artificial joints or partial limb amputations should be tested.

0 = No drift – The patient is able to hold the outstretched limb for five seconds.

1 = Drift – the patient is able to hold the outstretched limb for five seconds but there is unsteadiness, fluttering, or drift of the limb.

2 = Some effort against gravity – the patient is unable to hold the outstretched limb for five seconds but there is some effort against gravity.

3 = No effort against gravity – the patient is not able to bring the limb off the bed but there is effort against gravity. If the limb is placed at the correct angle, the patient is unable to sustain the position.

4 = No movement – the patient is unable to move the limb. There is no effort against gravity.

9 = Untestable – may be used only if limb is missing or hip joint is fused.

7 Limb ataxia

This item is aimed at examining the patient for evidence of a unilateral cerebellar lesion. It will also detect limb movement abnormalities related to sensory or motor dysfunction. Limb ataxia is checked by the finger-to-nose and heel-to-shin tests. The physician should test the 'normal' side first. The movements should be well performed, smooth, accurate and non-clumsy. There should not be any dysmetria or dyssynergia. Non-verbal cues may be given to the patient. If a patient has dysmetria or dyssynergia in one limb, the score should be 1. If a patient has dysmetria or dyssynergia in both the arm and leg on one side, or if there are bilateral signs, the score should be 2. If limb ataxia is present, the ataxia should be rated as present regardless of the possible aetiology. This item may be scored 9 (untestable) only if there is complete paralysis of the limbs (Motor function score = 4), if the limb is missing, amputated, fused, or if the patient is comatose (1a level of consciousness = 3).

0 = Absent – the patient is able to perform both the finger-to-nose and heel-to-shin tasks well. The movements are smooth and accurate.

1 = Present unilaterally in either arm or leg – the patient is able to perform one of the two required tasks well.

2 = Present unilaterally in both arm and leg or bilaterally – the patient is unable to perform either task well. Movements are inaccurate, clumsy, or poorly done.

9 = Untestable – may be used only if Motor function score = 4, limb is missing, amputated or fused, or if item 1a level of consciousness = 3.

8 Sensory

The patient is examined with a pin in the proximal portions of all four limbs and asked how the stimulus feels. The patient's eyes do not need to be closed. The patient is asked if the stimulus is sharp or dull and if there is any asymmetry between the right and left sides. Only sensory loss that can be attributed to stroke should be counted as abnormal – usually this will be a hemisensory loss. Sensory loss due to a non stroke-related condition, such as a neuropathy, should not be graded as abnormal. If a patient has depressed level of consciousness, neglect, aphasia or is unable to describe the sensory perception, the patient's non-verbal responses, such as a grimace or withdrawal, should be graded. If the patient responds to the stimulus, it should be scored 0. The response to the stimulus on the right and left sides should be compared. If the patient does not respond to a noxious stimulus on one side, the score should be 2. Patients with severe depression of consciousness should be examined.

0 = Normal – no sensory loss to pin is detected.

1 = Partial loss – mild to moderate diminution in perception to pin stimulation is recognized. This may involve more than one limb.

2 = Dense loss – severe sensory loss so that the patient is not aware of being touched. Patient does not respond to noxious stimuli applied to that side of the body.

9 Best language

The patient's language will be tested by having the patient identify standard groups of objects and by reading a series of sentences. Comprehension of language should be judged as the physician performs the entire neurologic examination. The physician should give the patient adequate time to identify the objects on the sheet of paper, see page 97. Only the first response is measured. If the patient misidentifies the object and later corrects him/herself, the response is still considered abnormal. The physician should then give the patient a sheet of paper with a series of sentences, see below. The examiner should ask the patient to read at least three sentences.

The first attempt to read the sentence is measured. If the patient misreads the sentence and later corrects him/herself the response is still considered abnormal. If the patient's visual loss precludes visual identification of objects or reading, the examiner should ask the patient to identify objects placed in his/her hand and the examiner should judge the patient's spontaneous speech and ability to repeat sentences. If the examiner judges these responses as normal the score should be 0. If the patient is intubated or is unable to speak, the examiner should check the patient's writing.

0 = No aphasia – the patient is able to read the sentences well and is able to correctly name the objects on the sheet of paper.

1 = Mild to moderate aphasia – the patient has mild to moderate naming errors, word finding errors, paraphasias or mild impairment in comprehension or expression.

2 = Severe aphasia – the patient has severe aphasia with difficulty in reading as well as naming objects. Patient with either Broca's (expressive) or Wernicke's (receptive) aphasia are included here.

3 = Mute.

Reading sentences for best language item in NIH stroke scale:

- You know how.
- Down to earth.
- I got home from work.
- Near the table in the dining room.
- They heard him speak on the radio last night.

10 Dysarthria

The primary method of examination is to ask the patient to read and pronounce a standard list of words from a sheet of paper, see page 98. If the patient is unable to read the words because of visual loss, the physician may say the word and ask the patient to repeat it. If the patient has severe aphasia, the clarity of articulation of spontaneous speech should be

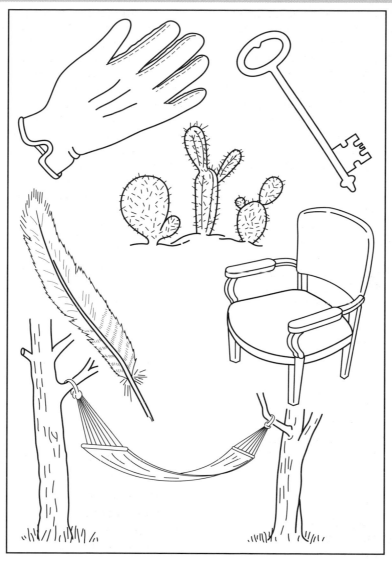

Images to be identified in best language item in NIH stroke scale.

rated. If the patient is mute or comatose (item 9 best language = 3) or has an endotracheal tube, this item can be rated as 9 (untestable).

0 = Normal articulation – patient is able to pronounce the words clearly and without any problem in articulation.

1 = Mild to moderate dysarthria – patient has problems in articulation. Mild to moderate

slurring of words is noted. The patient can be understood but with some difficulty.

2 = Near unintelligible or worse – patient's speech is so slurred that it is unintelligible.

9 = Untestable – may be used only if item 9 best language = 3, or if the patient has an endotracheal tube.

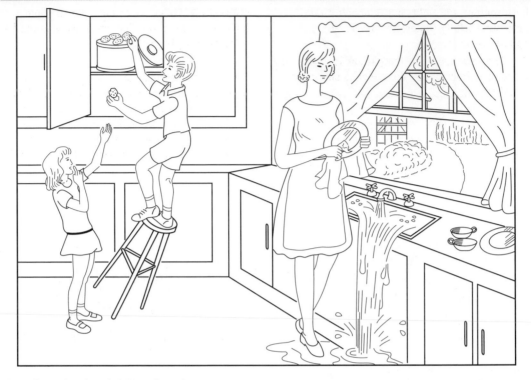

Picture for neglect item in NIH stroke scale.

Words for dysarthria item in NIH stroke scale:

- mama
- tip-top
- fifty–fifty
- thanks
- huckleberry
- baseball player
- caterpillar

11 Neglect (extinction and inattention)

The presence of neglect is examined by the patient's ability to recognize simultaneous cutaneous sensory and visual stimuli from the right and left sides. The visual stimulus is a standard picture. The picture is shown to the patient and she/he is asked to describe it. The physician should encourage the patient to scan the picture and identify features on both the right and left sides of the picture. The physician should encourage the patient to compensate for any visual loss. If the patient does not identify parts of the picture on one side, the result should be considered abnormal. The physician then assesses the ability to recognize bilateral simultaneous touch to upper or lower limbs. The test is done by touching the patient when the patient's eyes are closed. The test should be considered abnormal if the patient ignores sensory stimuli from one side of the body. If the patient has a severe visual loss and the cutaneous stimuli are normal, the score should be 0. If the patient has aphasia and is unable to describe the picture, but does attend to both sides, the score should be 0.

0 = No neglect – the patient is able to recognize bilateral simultaneous cutaneous stimuli on the right and left sides of the body and is able to identify images on the right and left sides of the picture.

1 = Partial neglect – the patient is able to recognize either cutaneous or visual stimuli on

both the left and right, but is unable to do both successfully (unless severe visual loss or aphasia is present).

2 = Complete neglect – the patient is unable to recognize either bilateral cutaneous sensory or visual stimuli.

Unified neurological stroke scale

The unified stroke scale takes elements from the Scandinavian stroke scale (SNSS) and the Orgogozo neurological score. Unlike the NIH stroke scale, these scales are used to grade hand motor function. The worst score would be 0 for each of these scales.

Other stroke neurological assessment scales based on impairments are available, including the Canadian Neurological Scale, Mathew Scale, Stroke Data Bank score, Italian Stroke Scale, European Stroke Scale, Allen score and other clinical neurology examination schemes used in published studies.

Unified neurological stroke scale			
Item	Unified	SNSS	Orgogozo
Consciousness			
Normal – fully conscious	4	6	15
Somnolent/drowsiness	3	4	10
Reacts to verbal command	2	2	10
Stupor (reacts to pain only)	1	0	5
Speech/verbal communication			
Normal/no aphasia	3	10	10
Limited vocabulary or incoherent speech/difficult	2	6	5
More than yes–no but no longer sentences/difficult	1	3	5
Only yes–no or less/extremely difficult or impossible	0	0	0
Eye movements/eyes and head shift			
No gaze palsy/none	2	4	10
Gaze palsy or gaze failure	1	2	5
Conjugate eye deviation/forced	0	0	0
Facial palsy			
None/dubious/slight paresis	1	2	5
Present, paralysis or marked paresis	0	0	0
Arm motor			
Raises with normal strength	4	6	10
Raises with reduced strength (possible)	3	5	10
Raises with flexion in elbow (incomplete)	2	4	5
Can move but not against gravity/impossible	1	2	0
Paralysis	0	0	0
Hand motor			
Normal strength	3	6	15
Reduced strength (skilled movements)	2	4	10
Fingertips do not reach palms (useful)	1	2	5
Paralysis (useless)	0	0	0
Upper limb tone			
Normal (even if brisk reflexes)	1	–	5
Overtly spastic or flaccid	0	–	0

continued

continued

Leg motor

Raises with normal strength	4	6	15
Raises with reduced strength (against resistance)	3	5	10
Raises with flexion in knee (against gravity)	2	4	5
Can move but not against gravity/impossible	1	2	0
Paralysis	0	0	0

Foot dorsiflexion

Against resistance/normal	2	–	10
Against gravity	1	–	5
Foot drop	0	–	0

Lower limb tone

Normal (even if brisk reflexes)	1	–	5
Overtly spastic or flaccid	0	–	0

Orientation

Correct for time, place and person	3	6	–
Two of three	2	4	–
One of three	1	2	–
Completely disorientated	0	0	–

Gait

Walks at least five metres without aids	4	12	–
Walk with aids	3	9	–
Walk with help of another person	2	6	–
Sits without support	1	3	–
Bedridden/wheelchair	0	0	–
TOTAL	**0–32**	**0–58**	**0–100**

Barthel index

The Barthel index contains 10 items that measure daily functioning, specifically the activities of daily living (ADL) and mobility. The items include feeding, moving from wheelchair to bed and return (if appropriate), grooming, transferring to and from a toilet, bathing, walking, going up and down stairs, dressing and continence. The assessment can be used to determine a baseline level of functioning and can be used to monitor improvement in activities of daily living over time. The items are weighted according to a scheme developed by the authors of a paper published in 1965. The person is assigned a score based on whether they have received help while doing the task or not. The scores for each item are summed to create a total score. The higher the score, the more 'independent' the person. Independence means that the person needs no assistance at any part of the task.

In some versions of the index 0, 1, 2 and 3 are used to replace 0, 5, 10 and 15. (We have reproduced the original version.) It should be scored carefully – it should be used as a record of what a patient does, not what a patient could do. The main aim is to establish the degree of independence by monitoring all help, physical or verbal, however minor and for whatever reason. The need for supervision renders the patient not independent. Middle categories imply that the patient supplies over 50% of the effort. Use of aids to be independent is allowed. A patient's performance should be established using the best available evidence. Asking questions to the patient, their friends/relatives and nurses are the usual sources of information, but direct observation and common sense are also important. However, direct testing is not essential – usually the patient's performance over the past 24–48 hours is important, but occasionally longer periods will be relevant.

Barthel index

Activity	Score			
Bowels 0 = incontinent (or needs to be given enemas) 5 = occasional accident 10 = continent	0	5	10	
Bladder 0 = incontinent or catheterized and unable to manage alone 5 = occasional accident 10 = continent	0	5	10	
Grooming 0 = needs help with personal care 5 = independent face/hair/teeth/shaving (implements provided)	0	5		
Toilet use 0 = dependent 5 = needs some help but can do something alone 10 = independent (on and off, dressing, wiping)	0	5	10	
Feeding 0 = unable 5 = needs help cutting, spreading butter, etc. or requires modified diet 10 = independent	0	5	10	
Transfers (bed to chair and back) 0 = unable, no sitting balance 5 = major help (one or two people, physical), can sit 10 = minor help (verbal or physical) 15 = independent	0	5	10	15
Mobility (on level surfaces) 0 = immobile or < 50 yards 5 = wheelchair independent, including corners, >50 yards 10 = walks with help of one person (verbal or physical) >50 yards 15 = independent (but may use an aid, eg a walking stick) >50 yards	0	5	10	15
Dressing 0 = dependent 5 = needs help but can do about half unaided 10 = independent (including buttons, zips, laces, etc.)	0	5	10	
Stairs 0 = unable 5 = needs help (verbal, physical, carrying aid) 10 = independent	0	5	10	
Bathing 0 = dependent 5 = independent (or in shower)	0	5		

Total (0–100)

The Barthel index is a useful index of recovery. It does suffer from a 'plateau effect' – even when recovery is incomplete it is possible to obtain the maximum score.

Modified Rankin scale

The modified Rankin scale is widely used to grade handicap. It should be used to estimate the degree of handicap before the stroke occurred and during rehabilitation and follow-up. The original Rankin scale was first published in 1957 and has been slightly modified by Warlow and associates for the UK-TIA study to accommodate language disorders and cognitive defects: the original scale did not contain Grade 0, defined Grade 1 as 'no significant disability: able to carry out all usual duties', and defined Grade 2 as 'slight disability: unable to carry out some of the previous activities . . .'.

Instrumental activities of daily living

The Lawton instrumental activities of daily living (IADL) scale is easy to use. The IADL assessment scale allows a health professional to establish the levels at which an elderly individual functions in caring for himself or herself and performs the more sophisticated tasks of everyday life. The evaluator sets standards appropriate to the clinical situation for determining if the person is doing well, formulating a treatment plan and arranging appropriate treatment and services.

A patient is awarded two points for each area in which he/she can function totally without help, one point in those areas that they need some help and no points for those activities that somebody else must do completely for them. The maximum score is 16 and the minimum score is zero.

Modified Rankin scale	
Grade 0	No symptoms at all
Grade 1	No significant disability despite symptoms: able to carry out all usual duties and activities
Grade 2	Slight disability: unable to carry out all previous activities but able to look after affairs without assistance
Grade 3	Moderate disability: requiring some help, but able to walk without assistance
Grade 4	Moderately severe disability: unable to walk without assistance and unable to attend to own bodily needs
Grade 5	Severe disability: bedridden, incontinent and requiring constant nursing care and attention
Grade 6	Dead

IADL			
Activity	Needs no help (2 points each)	Needs some help (1 point each)	Unable to do at all (0 points each)
1. Using the telephone	___	___	___
2. Getting to places beyond walking distance	___	___	___
3. Grocery shopping	___	___	___
4. Preparing meals	___	___	___
5. Doing housework or handyman work	___	___	___
6. Doing laundry	___	___	___
7. Taking medications	___	___	___
8. Managing money	___	___	___
Total score: ___ =	(___ × 2 =) ___ +	(___ × 1=) ___ +	0

Like other evaluations, the IADL scale provides a baseline of data that can be compared with the results of future evaluations. (Note that some activities may be gender specific. Omit these items if the patient does not usually perform those tasks.)

Geriatric depression scale

The geriatric depression scale can be used to evaluate elderly individuals for depressive symptoms. It is a self-rating instrument that is easy to answer and is geared towards the geriatric patient.

- 'No' answers are considered depressive responses in questions 1, 5, 7, 9, 15, 19, 21, 27, 29 and 30.

- 'Yes' answers are considered depressive responses in questions 2, 3, 4, 6, 8, 10, 11, 12, 13, 14, 16, 17, 18, 20, 22, 23, 24, 25, 26 and 28.

The total score = sum of points for all 30 questions.

Interpretation

The results should be interpreted with discretion:

- scores of 0–10 are not increased and are 'normal' for the elderly
- scores of 11–13 are borderline
- scores of 14–30 are increased and associated with depression.

Geriatric depression scale

	Choose the best answer for how you felt over the past week	Yes	No
		Points for response	
1	Are you basically satisfied with your life?	0	1
2	Have you dropped many of your activities and interests?	1	0
3	Do you feel that your life is empty?	1	0
4	Do you often get bored?	1	0
5	Are you hopeful about the future?	0	1
6	Are you bothered by thoughts you can't get out of your head?	1	0
7	Are you in good spirits most of the time?	0	1
8	Are you afraid that something bad is going to happen to you?	1	0
9	Do you feel happy most of the time?	0	1
10	Do you often feel helpless?	1	0
11	Do you often get restless and fidgety?	1	0
12	Do you prefer to stay at home, rather than going out and doing new things?	1	0
13	Do you frequently worry about the future?	1	0
14	Do you feel you have more problems with memory than most?	1	0
15	Do you think it is wonderful to be alive now?	0	1
16	Do you often feel downhearted and blue?	1	0
17	Do you feel pretty worthless the way you are now?	1	0
18	Do you worry a lot about the past?	1	0
19	Do you find life very exciting?	0	1
20	Is it hard for you to get started on new projects?	1	0
21	Do you feel full of energy?	0	1
22	Do you feel that your situation is hopeless?	1	0
23	Do you think that most people are better off than you are?	1	0
24	Do you frequently get upset over little things?	1	0
25	Do you frequently feel like crying?	1	0
26	Do you have trouble concentrating?	1	0
27	Do you enjoy getting up in the morning?	0	1
28	Do you prefer to avoid social gatherings?	1	0
29	Is it easy for you to make decisions?	0	1
30	Is your mind as clear as it used to be?	0	1

MRC clinical grading scale

Abnormalities of reflexes are commonly seen in stroke patients. The MRC clinical grading scale for tendon reflexes is outlined below:

- – = not present
- +/– = present with reinforcement
- + = present
- ++ = obviously present
- +++ = brisk
- ++++ = pathologically brisk with clonus.

Further reading

Bonita R, Beaglehole R. Recovery of motor function after stroke. *Stroke* 1988; **19**: 1497–500.

Collin C, Wade DT, Davis S, Horne V. The Barthel ADL Index: a reliability study. *Int Disabil Stud* 1988; **10**: 61–3.

Lawton MP. Instrumental Activities of Daily Living (IADL) Scale. Self-rated version. Incorporated in the Philadelphia Geriatric Center. Multilevel Assessment Instrument (MAI). *Psychopharmacol Bull* 1998; **24(4)**: 789–91.

Mahoney FI, Barthel D. Functional evaluation: the Barthel Index. *Md State Med J* 1965; **14**: 56–61.

Multicenter trial of hemodilution in ischemic stroke – background and study protocol. Scandinavian Stroke Study Group. *Stroke* 1985; **16**: 885–90.

Orgogozo JM, Capildeo R, Anagnostou CN *et al*. Development of a neurological score for clinical evaluation of sylvian infarctions. *Presse Med* 1983; **12(48)**: 3039–44.

Rankin J. Cerebral vascular accidents in patients over the age of 60. *Scott Med J* 1957; **2**: 200–15.

Van Swieten JC, Koudstaal PJ, Visser MC *et al*. Interobserver agreement for the assessment of handicap in stroke patients. *Strokep* 1988; **19**: 604–7.

Index

Page number is *italics* refer to information that is shown only in a table or diagram.